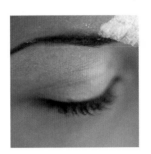

Ann Redfearn

Insomnia

Take control of your health naturally

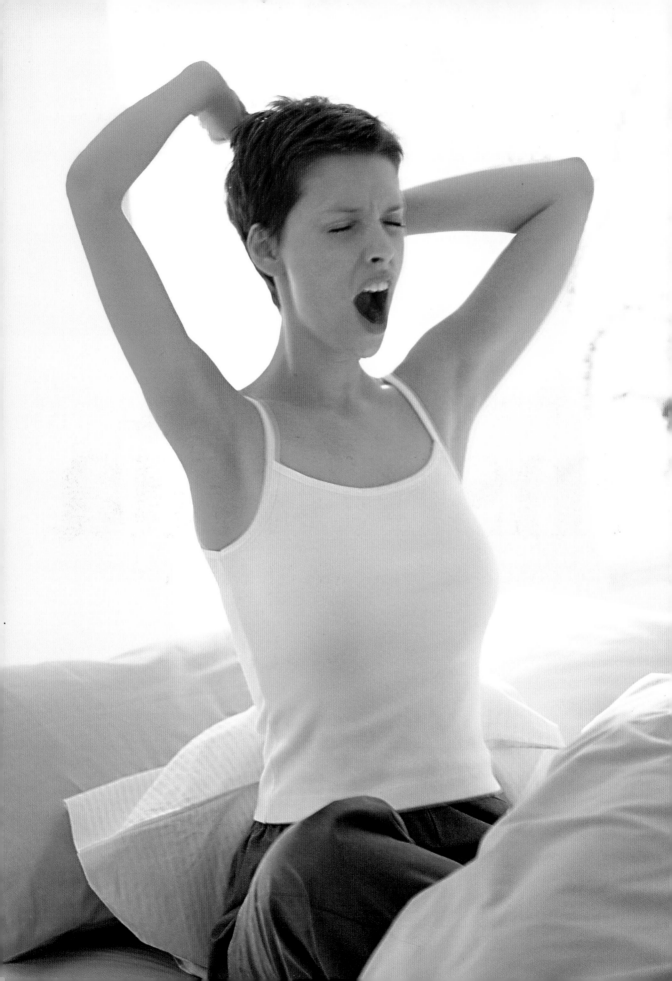

GAIA HOLISTIC HEALTH SERIES

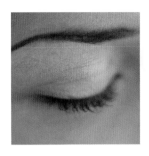

Ann Redfearn

Insomnia

Take control of your health naturally

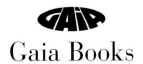

Gaia Books

Project Editor Kelly Thompson
Design Phil Gamble
Photography Ruth Jenkinson, Dave King,
Direction Jo Godfrey Wood, Patrick Nugent

® This is a Registered Trade Mark of Gaia Books

First published in 2005 in the United Kingdom by:
Gaia Books, an imprint of Octopus Publishing Group Ltd
2–4 Heron Quays, Canary Wharf, London E14 4JP

Text © Ann Redfearn 2005
Illustrations and compilation © Gaia Books 2005

A CIP catalogue record for this book is available from
the British library:

ISBN: 1-85675-234-8
EAN: 9 781856 752343

Distributed in the United States and Canada by
Sterling Publishing Co., Inc., 387 Park Avenue South, New York, NY 10016–8810

Manufactured in China

10 9 8 7 6 5 4 3 2 1

Author photograph: Peter Carrick

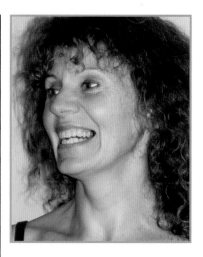

Author: Ann Redfearn BSY (DS, Arom, Col)

Ann is a qualified tai chi and kai men (Chinese Yoga) instructor, who has been studying and teaching for seventeen years. She is also a qualified aroma-therapist, colour therapist, holistic diagnostician, and feng shui practitioner. Her experience has led to an awareness of and sensitivity to the human energy field and through this she has developed a range of varying natural healing techniques – in the knowledge that different people have different needs, changing and developing over time. Ann hopes that a wider audience might benefit as much as she, her friends, her family, and her clients have done over the years.

Contents

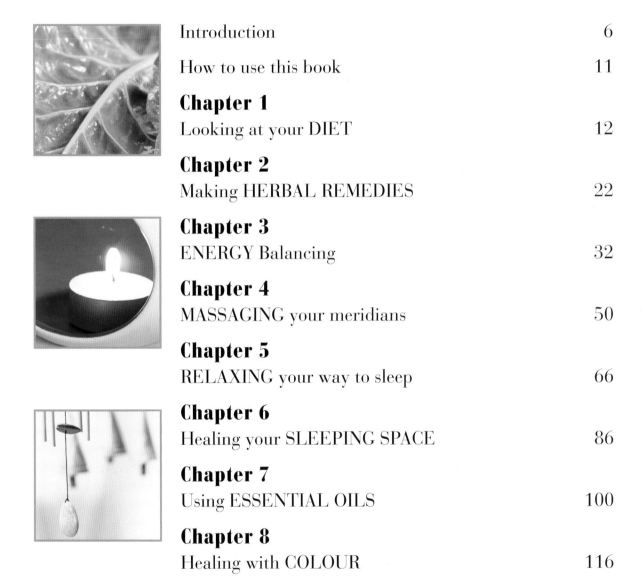

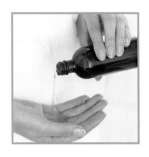

Disclaimer

The information and exercises given in this book are in no way intended to replace professional medical advice. Neither the author nor the publishers shall be liable nor responsible for any loss, injury, or damage allegedly arising from any information or suggestion in this book.

Introduction

Insomnia is one of the scourges of modern society. In addition to the long, lonely hours spent lying in bed wide awake but exhausted, there can be huge effects on the quality of sufferers' daytime hours due to a lack of energy and a general sense of not being able to cope.

The number of people being affected by insomnia is on the increase. Present figures show that a staggering 40 percent of women and 30 percent of men in the Western world are seeking help in order to cope with it. And that doesn't include those suffering in silence.

Importance of sleep

Good-quality sleep is an essential ingredient of a healthy life as it provides time for our mind to process the preceding day's activities (often in the form of dreams) and for our body to rejuvenate, repair, and heal itself. It is also time for our energy to realign and rebalance itself – particularly during times of distress or emotional overload. Sleep therefore forms a part of our natural cycle, and a lack of it can result in continuous feelings of nervousness, being out of control, and a complete inability to relax, make sound decisions, or function "normally".

During regular, restful sleep, the blood pressure naturally falls – preventing such problems as hypertension – but during periods of sleeplessness and disturbance, this natural process is interrupted. It is also thought that insufficient sleep can interfere with hormone production, in particular those related to weight gain, which makes a balanced diet all the more important (see pp. 14–17).

Sleep requirements

The amount of sleep you require varies throughout life, and one person's needs will be vastly different from another's. A new-born baby will spend much of its time sleeping; a young child generally needs up to ten hours; a teenager often needs around

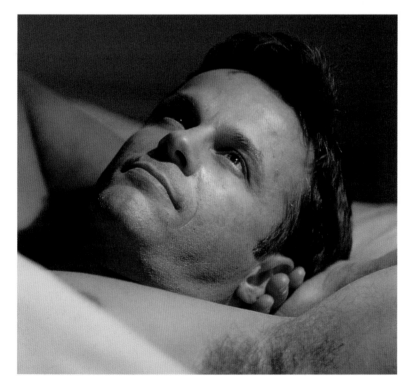

DOG TIRED
There's nothing worse than lying awake at night, feeling there's nothing you can do to help yourself get back to sleep.

personal life force, such
as by healthy eating
habits, regular exercise,
relaxation time, and positive
states of mind – as these all
contribute to "charging us up".
And this books aims to lead
you in the right direction in
all of these areas, and more.

Why insomnia?

There can't be many people
who do not have the occasional
disturbed night's sleep – it's
almost normal. The reason is
usually pretty apparent. Perhaps
it's because of pre-exam or pre-
interview nerves, or the excitement of a long-awaited event
fast approaching – such as your
wedding day or moving house –
or even as a result of an unusually
rich meal or strong coffee taken
late in the evening.

The trouble generally arises
when the sleeplessness is no
longer a one-off occurrence, but
becomes more routine. It may be
that you experience great
difficulty in dropping off to sleep
in the first place, your mind is
still racing from the day's
activities, or it may be that you
wake repeatedly or in the early
hours, and find it impossible to
get back to sleep again. You start
to turn things over in your mind,
darting from one perceived
problem to the next. Perhaps you

about eight or nine; and adults
tend to learn to do with less still.
However, research has shown
that people in non-industrialized
societies tend to sleep for around
ten hours, implying that our real
requirements are higher than we
allow in our pressurized lives.

It is therefore important to
be guided by your instinct about
what is right for you, regardless
of the unwritten rule that we all
need our eight hours. You may
well be different. Some people
find that they can cope with a
limited amount of sleep during
particularly busy periods of their
lives, being able to catch up at a
later point, when life quietens
down again. You may feel fine
and refreshed after only four or
five hours' sleep, while someone
else may feel unable to cope
effectively without eight, or
even nine, hours. It is only when
you are suffering as a result of
habitually not being able to get
as much sleep as you require
that you should actually feel
the need to seek treatment
for your insomnia – just as for
any other disorder.

Insomnia side effects

Insomnia sufferers are often left
feeling "on edge" and unable to
cope with the simplest of daily
tasks, and may experience a lack
of concentration, a decrease in
attention span, and/or a slowing
down of reactions. Not only can
these effects lead to anxiety and
depression, but they can also pose
serious health risks, such as when
driving or performing other
tasks that require the ability
to think clearly and rapidly.
Tempers may flare and family
relationships may feel the strain,
as there is little energy left for
leisure time. This leisure time is,
however, vital to overall health
as it increases personal energy,
or "life force" – the natural flow
of energy that permeates all
living things, ourselves included.
Ancient Chinese philosophy
teaches that when this force is
flowing well, health and balance
ensue, and that when it is not, a
lack of well-being is experienced
– through myriad physical
symptoms, insomnia included.

There are many ways in which
we can seek to improve our

spend a couple of hours tossing and turning, only to fall asleep exhausted when it is almost time for the alarm to sound. The minutes tick away, turning into hours, while the whole world seems – annoyingly – to be blissfully slumbering. But here you are, wide awake, knowing your stressful day is looming closer, and wondering, again, just how you're going to cope. The irony is that the more you think about it and the more anxious you become, the less likely you are to get back to sleep.

Trust that when the time is right, circumstances will prevail to prompt change

Increasingly, sleeplessness is caused by this type of underlying stress – unresolved worries and emotions, which have a nasty habit of making themselves known to you in the dead of night, leaving you with a racing pulse and a head full of whirling, anxiety-provoking thoughts. Not

a good recipe for peaceful and restorative sleep. These feelings of responsibility, and demands on our time and conscience, end up not only stressing the mind, but also overloading the body. It literally feels as though it is "under attack" and has to take emergency action to cope with

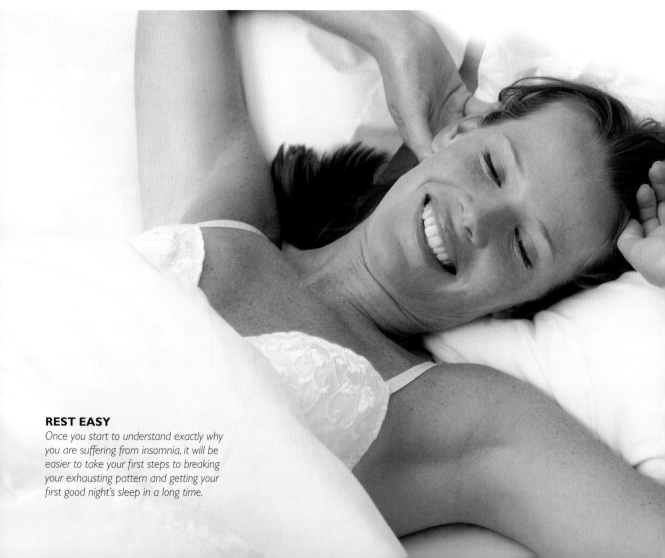

REST EASY
Once you start to understand exactly why you are suffering from insomnia, it will be easier to take your first steps to breaking your exhausting pattern and getting your first good night's sleep in a long time.

the brain's stress signals. One example of this is an increase in adrenaline production ("fight or flight" syndrome), which in turn makes relaxation and sleep all the more out of reach.

The pressure's on

Perhaps, then, the frequent inability to get to sleep, and stay asleep, is a negative by-product of our twenty-four-hour, seven-days-a-week world, in which we constantly aim to beat the clock. After all, the chaotic lifestyles we lead often seem to proceed at such a pace that we feel that we have in some way failed if we are unable to keep up, or if we become exhausted or disillusioned. It seems as though we never really get the chance to relax properly – switch off, unplug ourselves, and remove the batteries – day or night. Is it because we don't dare to, haven't effectively learned how to, or have even "forgotten" how to? Or is it because society makes us feel driven to push ourselves until we drop?

The many pressures that modern-day lifestyles impose on us, such as long working hours, tight deadlines, and the constant need to be "on call" – whether by phone, e-mail, or text – have had the result of removing us from a more natural way of being. Whereas we previously had a clear distinction between day and night,

which enabled us to have periods of activity followed by periods of rest, we have largely removed these forces of nature from our lives. Instead, society seeks to produce one constant, artificial daytime, and as far as possible, one constant season – regulated by means of artificial heating and air conditioning. It is little wonder that our nervous systems are under so much strain and our mechanisms for sleep and renewal have been disrupted. As a result of almost constant overstimulation our poor nerves are never given a chance to rest.

We must therefore make a conscious effort to find ways of bringing a more natural balance into our lives – habits that nourish and nurture us. Otherwise, the artificial reality of the modern world threatens to immerse us in a soup of constant demands. It is up to each one of us to steer a path through this – to find a way which not only suits us, but which is conducive to continuing long-term good health. Sleep, or at the very least, good-quality rest, is one of the most essential ingredients, since without adequate recuperation time, the body can lose energy, and therefore the ability, to function normally, very quickly. We need to be brave enough to take time out when necessary – without guilt – in the knowledge that it is essential to our continued sanity, health, and well-being.

Time to look within

The inability to sleep sufficiently is indicative that time and effort must be spent to achieve balance once more in the body, as the body's needs have been pushed to one side – perhaps in deference to a constant stream of demands, or perhaps because you deny that you have any needs over and above what others expect of you? Sometimes, when we reach a crisis point, such as long-term sleeplessness, we are ready to make new, and perhaps drastic, decisions about ourselves, finally acknowledging that change is the only way forward. By opening this book you have already made the first step on this journey.

You may find you need a fundamental change of direction, in areas such as work and relationships, or you may find it's just a matter of a few simple dietary changes, alterations to your surroundings, or the introduction of gentle exercise, deeper breathing, or regular massage. Perhaps your diet (see pp. 14–17) is placing an already-tired body under strain by forcing it to use valuable energy to digest foods of limited nutritional value. Maybe your bed is uncomfortable, the bedroom too cluttered, your pillow too hard. Perhaps your lifestyle is too sedentary and you need to exercise more. Or maybe you are overactive, never really taking the time to relax completely.

Letting go

Alternatively, it may be that you don't allow any time to yourself, and that not sleeping has become, in a strange way, a method of spending time on your own. So take this opportunity to make a list of the demands on your time. List in one column the things that you enjoy and find fulfilling, and in the other all the demands that irritate you, overstretch you, or leave you feeling drained of energy. Now let go of certain demands that you place upon yourself, or that others place on you, remembering that a lack of energy toward something – or someone – is an internal sign that it may be either unnecessary, or even harmful, to you.

Although it takes a certain amount of courage, you need to recognize that the only way to regain the ability to sleep soundly is to implement change. We all have deep desires, and sometimes circumstances prevail until we are forced to make these dreams an important part of our lives. When this happens, and action is taken, people rarely look back. They find that they are suddenly fired up with a renewed energy for life, can sleep easy, and wonder why they couldn't find the impetus to take action before.

What to do

There are numerous sleeping pills available, some of which can prove very helpful. However, these are really only effective on a short-term basis – for example, during a relatively short-lived emotional crisis.

Much better for you in the long run are the many natural self-help techniques available, which – if used over a sustained

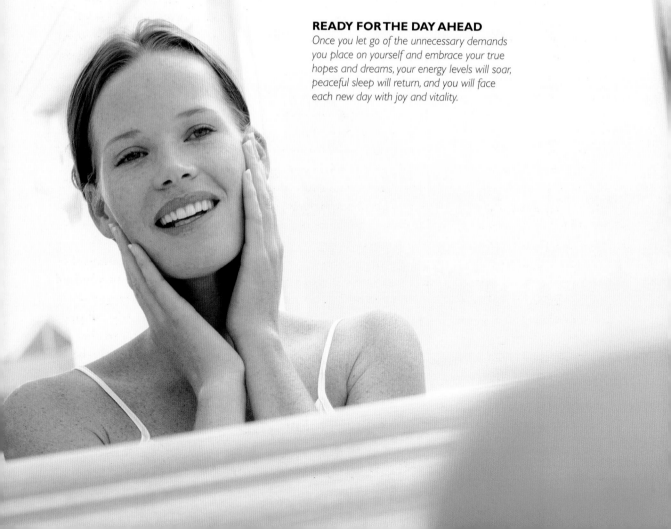

READY FOR THE DAY AHEAD
Once you let go of the unnecessary demands you place on yourself and embrace your true hopes and dreams, your energy levels will soar, peaceful sleep will return, and you will face each new day with joy and vitality.

period of time – should serve to improve your overall sense of well-being on a longer-term basis, increasing your energy levels during the day, and helping you sleep better at night.

This book encourages you to explore these natural means of rebalancing your life force. The aim is to bring you to a greater understanding of the internal and external factors affecting you, and to present you with simple methods of addressing them – for good. But as with all chronic conditions, it's also advisable to ask for a general health check from your doctor to see if he or she can help shed any light on the subject, too.

The techniques suggested are mostly based on ancient Chinese healing wisdom and many of them involve conscious relaxation as a way of freeing your mind, balancing your body, and encouraging quality rest.

You might try a delicious smoothie to help ease you into sleep, a soothing herbal tea or compress to help you unwind, aromatic oils to bring about a feeling of stillness, a self-massage to restore your energy balance, or a colour visualization to calm your spirit. Other areas explored are the "energy" in your sleeping environment – making use of Feng Shui wisdom – and breathing exercises, which can release the natural flow of life force and relax the mind and body enough for rest and sleep to take over.

How to use this book

This book takes you through a programme of self-help techniques, each one designed to teach you to "switch off" thoroughly from your busy life, to relax, and to get your mind, your body, and your spirit ready for a deep, restorative sleep.

You are free to choose the techniques that appeal to you most, which suit you best, and that really work for you as an individual, because everyone is different. You may want to work through the suggestions as they are presented, gradually developing your own awareness of which ones work best for you. Or you may have a strong urge to try particular techniques, and simply draw on others as your needs change. There are no hard and fast rules. And don't worry: although most of the techniques are inspired by Taoist principles – the philosophy behind the traditional Chinese healing arts – you will find them simple and easy to follow. The last thing you

want is to add to your stress levels with complicated rules and instructions, at a time when your energy is low to begin with.

Over time, you will develop a personal programme that works for you, giving rise to an improvement in the quality of your sleep and rest, and an increase in your overall feeling of well-being. This process of rebalancing will take some time, but the journey is a fulfilling one, and can lead you to a new depth of self-understanding. By teaching the mind and body how to relax and by educating your energy to work for you, not only will your quality of sleep improve, but your waking time will also be less exhausting.

Be guided by your innate wisdom, and enjoy the exploration

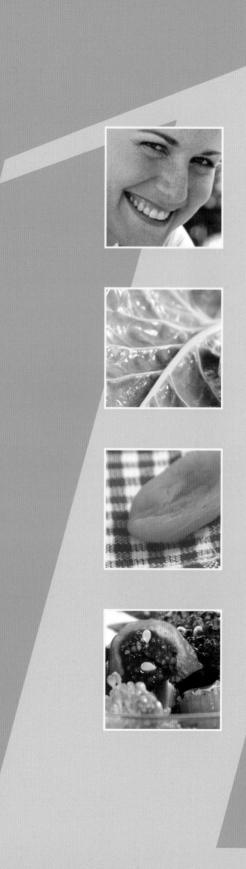

Chapter One

Looking at your
DIET

Taste the fruits of the garden

Drink from the fountain of life

We are what we eat

Most of us are familiar with the saying "we are what we eat": the idea that every single thing we consume provides a foundation on which we build our health. Yet few of us think carefully enough about the role that our food and drink play in creating bodily imbalances, which are often the cause of disturbances in our sleeping patterns.

The key point to remember is that if you eat a wide variety of nourishing foods and take the time to digest and assimilate them fully, your body will become stronger and more able to stave off any potential imbalances – restless sleep patterns included. However, there are also lots of specific dietary guidelines that can help you on your way to a healthier body, calmer mind, and improved sleeping patterns, and the following pages aim to outline some of these.

Avoid stimulants

As a first step, it's a good idea to look at and aim to decrease the amount of stimulants you take into your body (see box left for examples). These substances are really difficult for the body to process, which means that – far from providing the often sought-after pick-me-up – they actually put the body under great stress, undermining your ability to rest, relax, and rejuvenate.

"Junk" or "fast" food is the most obvious category of culprits.

Common Culprits

★ Tea & coffee
★ Chocolate
★ Fizzy drinks
★ Alcohol & nicotine
★ White sugar or products containing white sugar
★ Junk or fast food – hamburgers, beefburgers, french fries, pizzas, crisps, pre-prepared meals, tinned food, food high in artificial preservatives (the list goes on...)

Often, these sorts of foods boast long lists of additives, chemicals, and other suspect ingredients. If our diet contains a high quantity of such ingredients, the digestive system may feel the strain, leading to heartburn, indigestion, and constipation – all of which can severely disrupt quality sleep.

Another culprit of over-stimulation is refined, white sugar. Watch out on food labels for this as it often pops up in large quantities – not only in sweet snacks, but also in other more unexpected foods, such as pre-prepared and tinned foods. Its excessively stimulating effect on the body can lead to mood swings, fatigue, and loss of energy, thus disrupting the balance the body requires for sleep to occur. If you feel like sweetening yourself up, it's far better to do it with unrefined sugar, honey, or dried and fresh fruit.

Another top tip is to eliminate all sources of caffeine from your diet, at least for a while. Caffeine raises the heart rate, causes the breathing to become shallow, and overstimulates the adrenal glands, producing a stress reaction that contributes to the inability to sleep. It is therefore best to avoid drinking tea, coffee, chocolate-based drinks, colas, and any other caffeinated drinks, particularly toward the end of the day.

It is also a good idea to avoid alcohol and nicotine – both are stimulants that require a lot of vital energy to process. They therefore cause further stress to an already overloaded, sleep-deprived system. Although the occasional drink is not harmful, long-term and binge drinking are very detrimental to the major organs, leading to dehydration, irritation of the digestive processes, and irregularities in the heartbeat – all of which can contribute to wakefulness.

Lots of fruit & veg

It is common knowledge that regular fresh fruit and vegetables are crucial to a balanced diet, but few people know that certain fresh foods are thought to have a soporific effect on the body. Lettuce and dill seeds, for example, have both been known to have a sedating effect on the nervous system. Surprisingly, grapefruit juice has also been found helpful in promoting sleep, as have apples, apricots, and honey. Try blending a banana with grapefruit and apple juice for an evening drink, adding a

FEELING FRUITY

Regular consumption of a variety of fruits helps keep your body – and therefore your sleeping patterns – in balance.

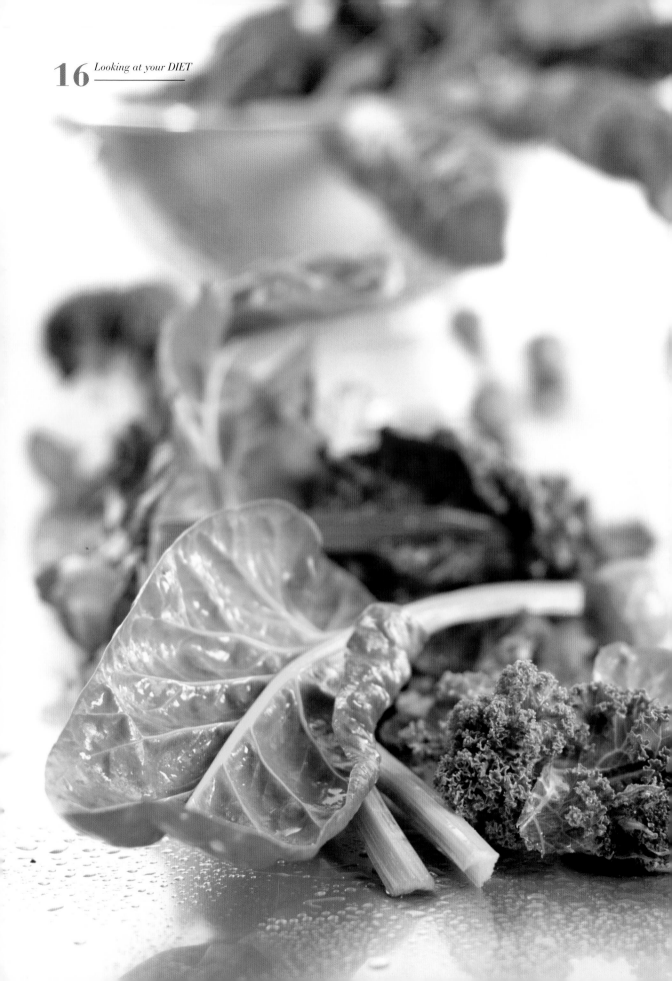

teaspoon of honey to taste if you want to add a sweetener. Alternatively, just try to incorporate some of these fruit and veg into your regular diet.

Vitamins and minerals

Chronic insomnia can often be linked to depression, anxiety, and other emotional upheavals, all of which cause a stress reaction and upset to the nervous system (see p. 9). It is therefore crucial to eat foods with a high vitamin B content. This nourishes the nervous system and can be found in leafy green vegetables, whole grains, nuts, seeds, eggs, fish, lean meat, wheat germ, and brewer's yeast.

However, it is also of crucial importance to include a plentiful supply of the other vitamins and minerals in your diet. Foods rich in vitamins A, B, C, and E can be particularly therapeutic for the adrenal glands, helping to control feelings of anxiety.

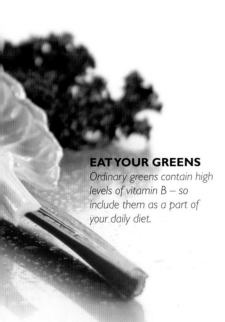

EAT YOUR GREENS
Ordinary greens contain high levels of vitamin B – so include them as a part of your daily diet.

GET YOUR OATS
Oats can be eaten in many forms and are a great source of vitamin B, which helps calm the nervous system.

Yellow fruits, vegetables, and oily fish are a good source of vitamin A, dark green vegetables and citrus fruits are rich in vitamin C, and vitamin E can be found in nuts, wheat germ, and vegetable oils.

Calming carbs

Try introducing a few daily portions of carbohydrates into your diet for their help in serotonin production. Serotonin is the "happiness" hormone, which is responsible for helping sleep regulation and reducing the tendency toward habitual worry and anxiety. Oats are especially good as they contain a wealth of B vitamins, as well as being high in carbs. Try hunting through cook books for recipes using oats and oatmeal to make delicious biscuits and cakes.

Calcium & Magnesium Boosters

★ Dairy products
★ Whole cereals
★ Wheat germ
★ Nuts & pulses
★ Sesame seeds
★ Watercress
★ Tinned sardines
★ Dried figs
★ Green vegetables – particularly broccoli and green cabbage

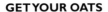

Oats can also be used instead of breadcrumbs in vegetable and cheese bakes. Other foods that help to promote serotonin production are apricots, bananas, honey, whole grains (organic if possible), and nuts.

Calcium & magnesium

It is also important to include foods in your diet that are rich in calcium and magnesium (see box, below left) as these minerals encourage healthy nerve function, helping to encourage the relaxation we need for sleep.

Timing

Get into the habit of eating your main meal at lunch-time rather than in the evening. If this is not possible, make sure you eat it at least three hours before bed, so that your digestive system is not working overtime when you retire. Try not to go to bed too hungry, as too little food causes that empty feeling, ensuring a restless night. Milk and chamomile tea can both help promote sleep: milk as it is rich in nerve-calming calcium, and chamomile as it helps prevent excess adrenaline from being produced.

Smoothies *juices* &

One of the very best ways of giving your body a real shot of what it needs, and loves – whether to help get you to sleep or improve your overall health – is to whizz up raw ingredients together in a blender. This way, you don't lose any of the vital nutrients that are usually lost, or diminished, during preparation and cooking, plus you get a delicious drink.

Benefits

As well as feeling like a real treat, smoothies and juices allow the body to use and assimilate nutrients much more rapidly than their component fruit and vegetables would, due to their liquid form. Consuming a variety of at least five servings per day of fruit and veg in this form can therefore quite quickly improve your underlying sense of well-being. This is because raw food not only provides vital nutrients that we can measure, but also gives us the nourishment of its vital life force, making us feel more healthy, energetic, and lively. Eating food in its raw state also gives the immune system a real boost because more of the natural nutrients are retained, making it a lot more difficult for colds, flu viruses, and other minor ailments to take hold.

Get blending

Try the recipe suggestions on the following pages or feel free to invent your own juicing and blending combinations. You might just want to use fruits and vegetables singly if you prefer more simple juices and smoothies or you can try an intriguing mix of sweet and savoury – it's entirely up to you. It is best to use organic produce wherever you possibly can in order to eliminate as many potentially harmful chemicals as you can from your intake. Wash the fruit and vegetables, peel them if appropriate, and blend them whole – pips, cores and all. The parts that people tend to throw away are often the bits that contain the most concentrated nutrients.

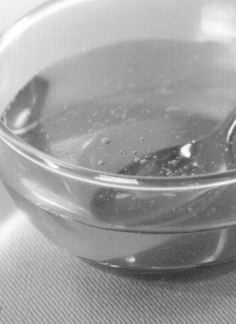

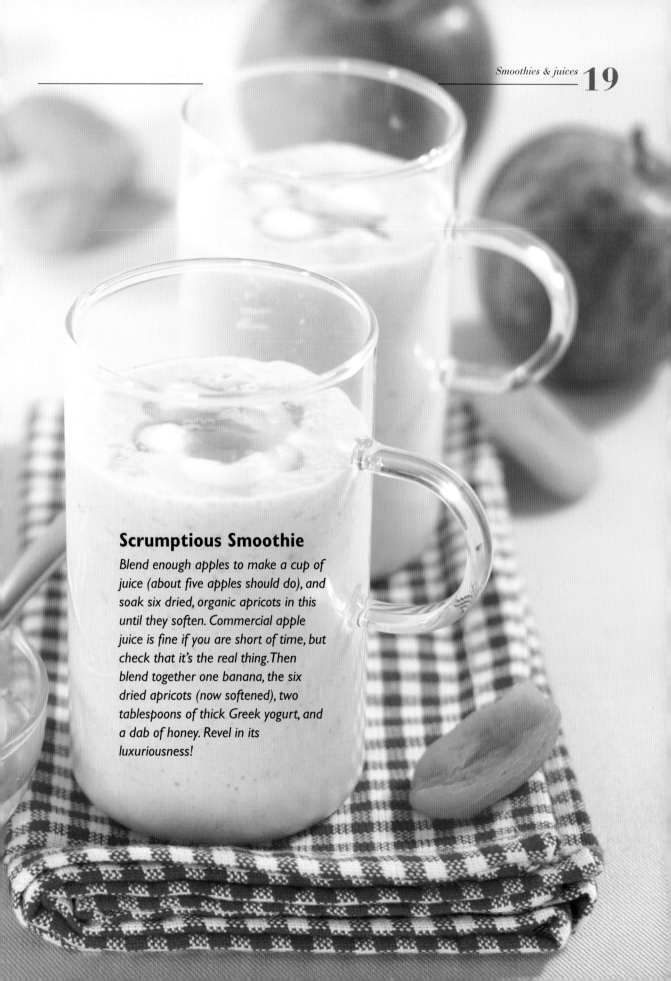

Scrumptious Smoothie

Blend enough apples to make a cup of juice (about five apples should do), and soak six dried, organic apricots in this until they soften. Commercial apple juice is fine if you are short of time, but check that it's the real thing. Then blend together one banana, the six dried apricots (now softened), two tablespoons of thick Greek yogurt, and a dab of honey. Revel in its luxuriousness!

Nerve Nourisher

Juice the following wonderful, health-giving ingredients together: approximately one part broccoli, one part watercress, one part parsley, three parts celery, and two parts spinach. Sip the resulting green juice slowly, letting your body receive deep nourishment and comfort from it.

...and if you don't have a juicer

If you don't have access to a juicer, you could finely chop the ingredients and eat them as a raw salad instead. Try adding chopped, dried figs and a sprinkling of sesame seeds for extra flavour. Sesame seeds also happen to be very rich in calcium. Garnish with a homemade dressing of lemon juice, olive oil, black pepper, and chopped basil — delicious!

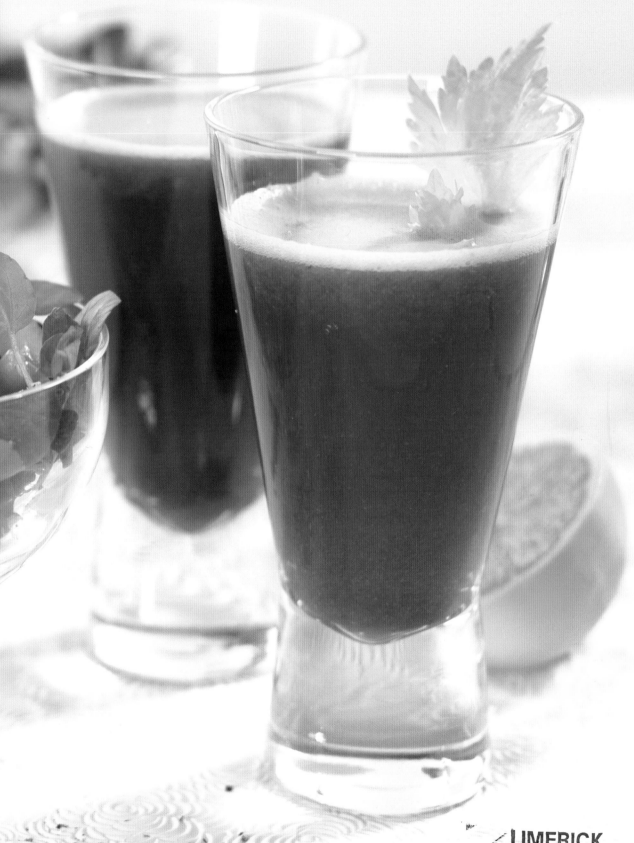

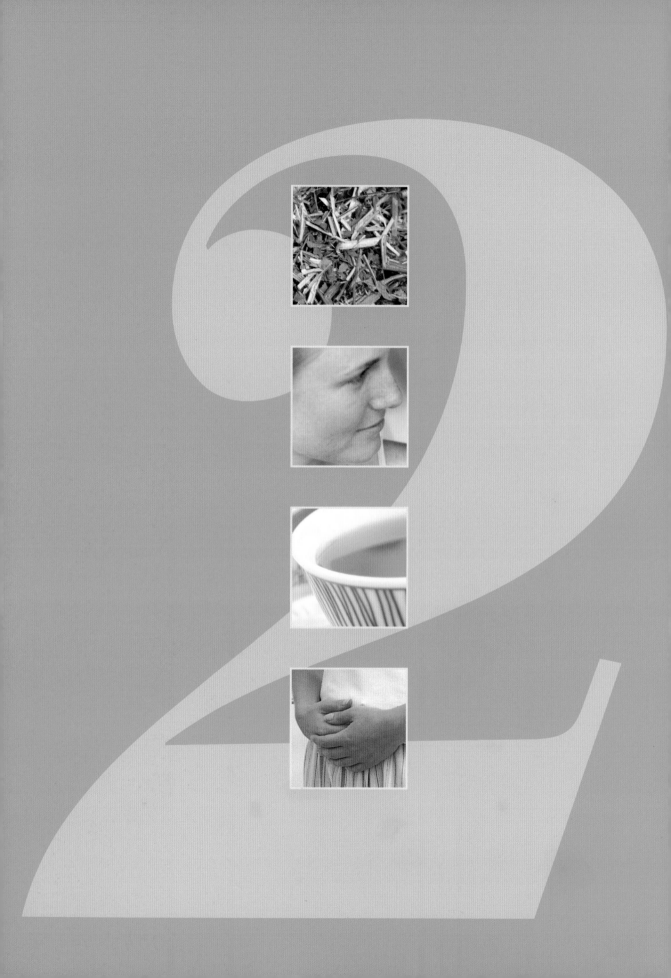

Chapter Two

Making

HERBAL
REMEDIES

Chamomile bids us to bed

Lavender calls distant dreams

Herbal *teas*

Herbal lore is the basis of an ancient healing system, which forms an important part of the traditional Chinese healing arts and is still in widespread use today. Quite a number of herbs – primarily chamomile, but also valerian, lime flowers, passiflora, hops, and St John's wort – are known to have a soothing effect on the nervous system in particular, and, for this reason, can be of substantial help in relieving insomnia.

Drinking teas made from a variety of therapeutic plants is an excellent way to let Mother Nature play her role in rebalancing your body and its patterns. The leaves of the plants should be used unless otherwise specified, and can be used dried or fresh, depending on availability. Most herbs should be available in local health food stores.

One-herb wonders
You can make a simple one-herb tea from any of the individual ingredients on the following pages, and you can even buy many of them in tea bag form these days. They make an ideal replacement drink for the times when you would previously have had a cup of normal tea or coffee – now that you're avoiding all caffeine, that is! And you can simply add honey to taste if you prefer a sweeter drink.

Herbs to help you sleep
Siberian Ginseng produces resistance to the effects of general stress, and calms nervous anxiety, restlessness, and emotional tension.
Asiatic Ginseng (in small doses) strengthens all the body's systems, increasing resistance to disease and improving efficiency in bodily functions.

Chamomile promotes a calm state of mind at times of stress and irritability.

As well as being useful in tea, chamomile can be used to make herb bags which can be placed under the pillow to aid sleep, in the same way as lavender bags are. Simply wrap a small piece of muslin (cheesecloth) around some chamomile and tie it up with ribbon or string.

Hops induces sleep, soothes headaches, and calms nervous disorders. In the 17th and 18th centuries, it became very popular to stuff pillows with hops in order to promote a restful night's sleep.

Basil clears the mind, helping to still unwanted thoughts. It is particularly therapeutic for exhaustion brought about by physical exertion.

St John's wort calms and strengthens the nerves, as well as bringing relief from irritability, anxiety, insomnia, and cramps.

Valerian relaxes muscular tension, lowers high blood pressure caused by nervousness, and considerably strengthens the nervous system.

Passiflora is deeply relaxing and sleep-inducing and has a beneficial effect on any muscular tension produced by excess anxiety.

Catnip is a great remedy for irritability and nerve-related headaches and insomnia.

Skullcap relieves irritability and decreases high blood pressure.

Lavender is a gentle tonic for the nervous and digestive systems. It is especially helpful in calming nervous anxiety, exhaustion, tension headaches, and depression.

Rose petals can be used to make a very soothing brew, which is of particular benefit for hormonal imbalances.

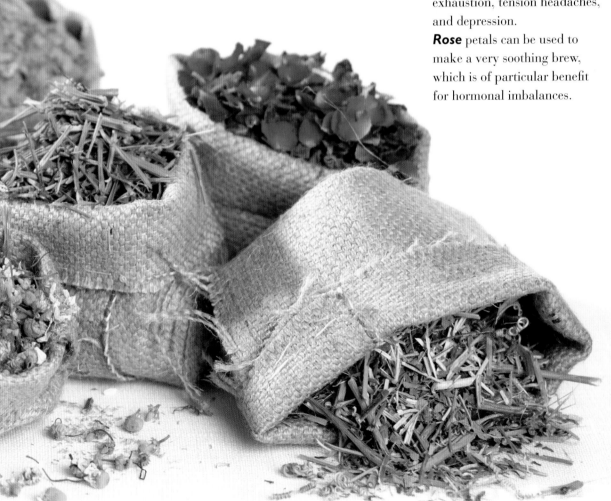

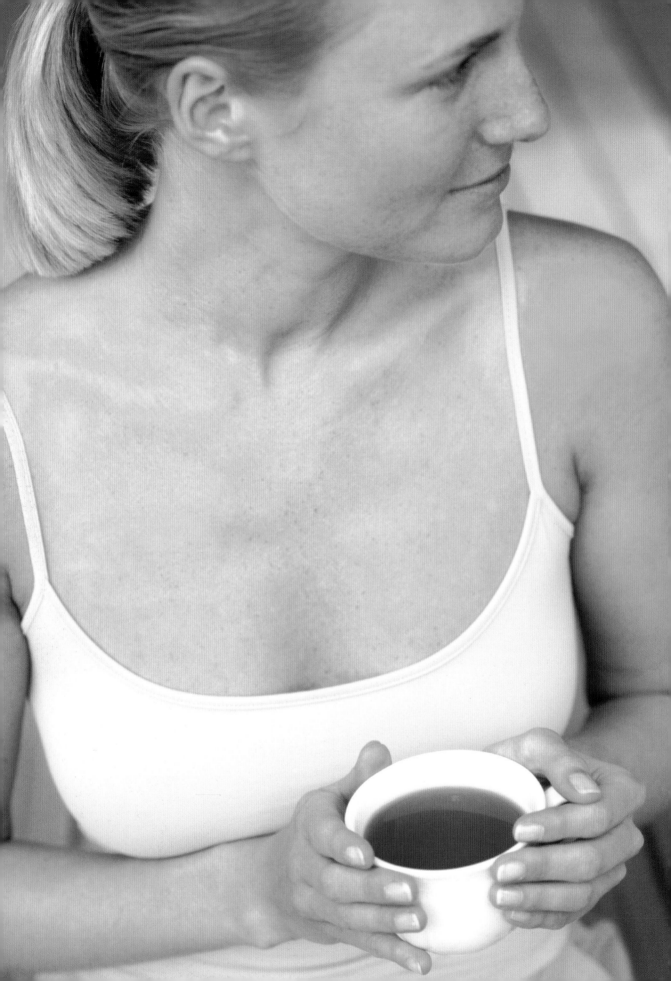

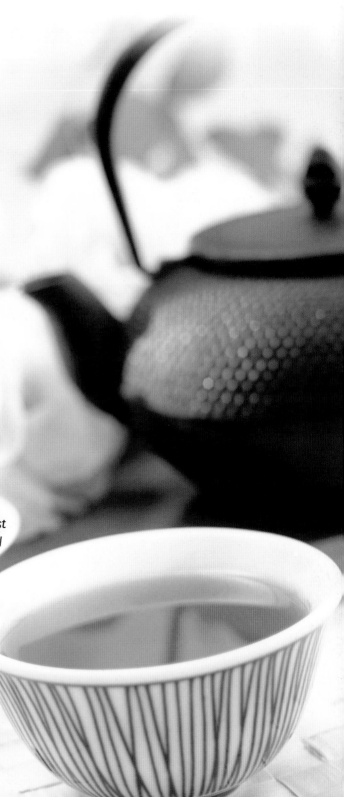

Goodnight Tea

Add a teaspoon of each of the following herbs to a litre (1 ¾pt) of boiling water: fresh peppermint, passiflora, chamomile, and valerian. Allow this mixture to infuse for twenty minutes in a covered container before straining it. Add honey to taste.

It is especially useful to sip your way through a warm cup of this about half an hour before going to bed.

Nerve Tonic

Add a teaspoon of each of the following herbs to a litre (1 ¾pt) of boiling water: celery seeds, catnip, valerian, and skullcap. Then add a teaspoon of vitamin B-rich oats, cover the container, and allow the mixture to infuse for twenty minute before straining it.

Sip one warm cup of this wonderfully relaxing tonic three times a day, between meals, and one in the evening before retiring. Or take when feeling anxious or "overcharged". The celery provides a delicious savoury flavour, but honey can be added if preferred.

Nerve Comforter

Add a teaspoon of each of the following to a litre (1 ¾pt) of boiling water: St John's wort, hops, basil, chamomile, and lime flowers. Allow the mixture to infuse for twenty minutes in a covered container before straining. Then add honey to taste.

Sip the warmed tea at intervals during the day, especially during moments of stress or anxiety, and just before going to bed. It is very beneficial for the adrenal glands – inhibiting the overproduction of adrenaline.

Ginseng Remedy

For a really potent tonic, simply add a teaspoon of Siberian or Asiatic ginseng to a cup of hot water. When taking ginseng, it's important to follow the guidelines on the packaging, indicating how much to take and how often, because this herb varies in strength according to the form in which you take it. Generally speaking, a low dose will act as a soother, while a large dose will act as a stimulant.

Herbal compresses

A compress is simply a wet or dry cloth which can be applied to some part of the body to relieve discomfort. We are all familiar with using an ice pack or a cold cloth for painful swellings, or perhaps a hot water bottle for an aching back.

In addition to the use of heat and cold, however, herbs can also be used to make compresses more effective. And when seeking relief from insomnia, herbs that provide healing, calming, or comforting properties are naturally the most useful. The best-known examples are chamomile and lavender, but ginger, too, has long been acknowledged as a healing herb, with its ability to warm, soothe, and energize. It acts as a general tonic by bringing comfort.

When to make a compress

You can make a hot compress very simply (see pp. 30–31) in order to relieve the inevitable side effects of insomnia, such as exhaustion and depleted energy. Most compresses should not be applied too late in the evening – never later than around two hours before bedtime. However, the ginger, chamomile, and lavender compresses on the following pages can be applied just before going to bed because of their soothing qualities.

Where to use your compresses

Oriental thinking tells us that the seat of our personal power and energy is found in an area known as the Tan Tien, or Lower Cauldron, which is located about 5cm (2in) below and behind the navel (see right). If you place your palms over this area on your stomach (see right), concentrate on it, and deepen your breathing toward it, you will precipitate energy flow and therefore hopefully experience a strong sense of this energy centre. This may be in the form of a slight tingling sensation or the spread of warmth beneath your hands.

Although compresses as we often know them (ice packs and the like) can be held almost

Turn inward for solace, letting the gentle fires of your innermost being bring you the comfort and peace you need

anywhere on the body, and lavender and chamomile ones are best held on the brow (see p. 31), the ginger compress should be held on the Tan Tien, as placing it elsewhere may prove too stimulating. Simply holding it over your Tan Tien will encourage energy to move into this area, where your body can easily use it when it needs it.

In Western culture our energy tends to be focused almost totally in the mind, which becomes frantically overactive, causing a depletion and imbalance of energy in the rest of the body. This is a major cause of disturbance in sleep patterns. The more your focus of attention can be encouraged down into the Tan Tien, the better it will be for the long-term health of your whole body, and the easier it will become to relax, restore energy, and finally get a good night's sleep.

When your focus is fully on your centre (the Tan Tien) your energy will start to flow in a balanced and strong way, and all your resources will be available to you as and when

you need them – whether to think and respond more clearly and quickly, to let go, to stop reacting in a destructive manner and just relax, or to get some undisturbed sleep for a change.

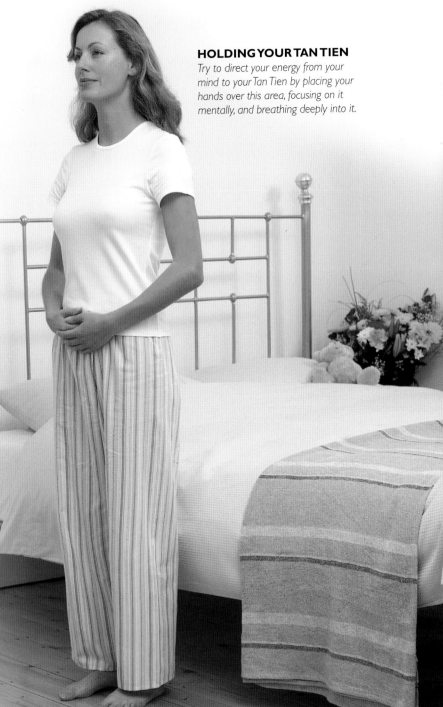

HOLDING YOUR TAN TIEN
Try to direct your energy from your mind to your Tan Tien by placing your hands over this area, focusing on it mentally, and breathing deeply into it.

5cm (2in)

LOCATING YOUR TAN TIEN
Your Tan Tien is the seat of your personal power and the centre of your energy according to Chinese healing philosophy. It is located approximately 5cm (2in) beneath the navel.

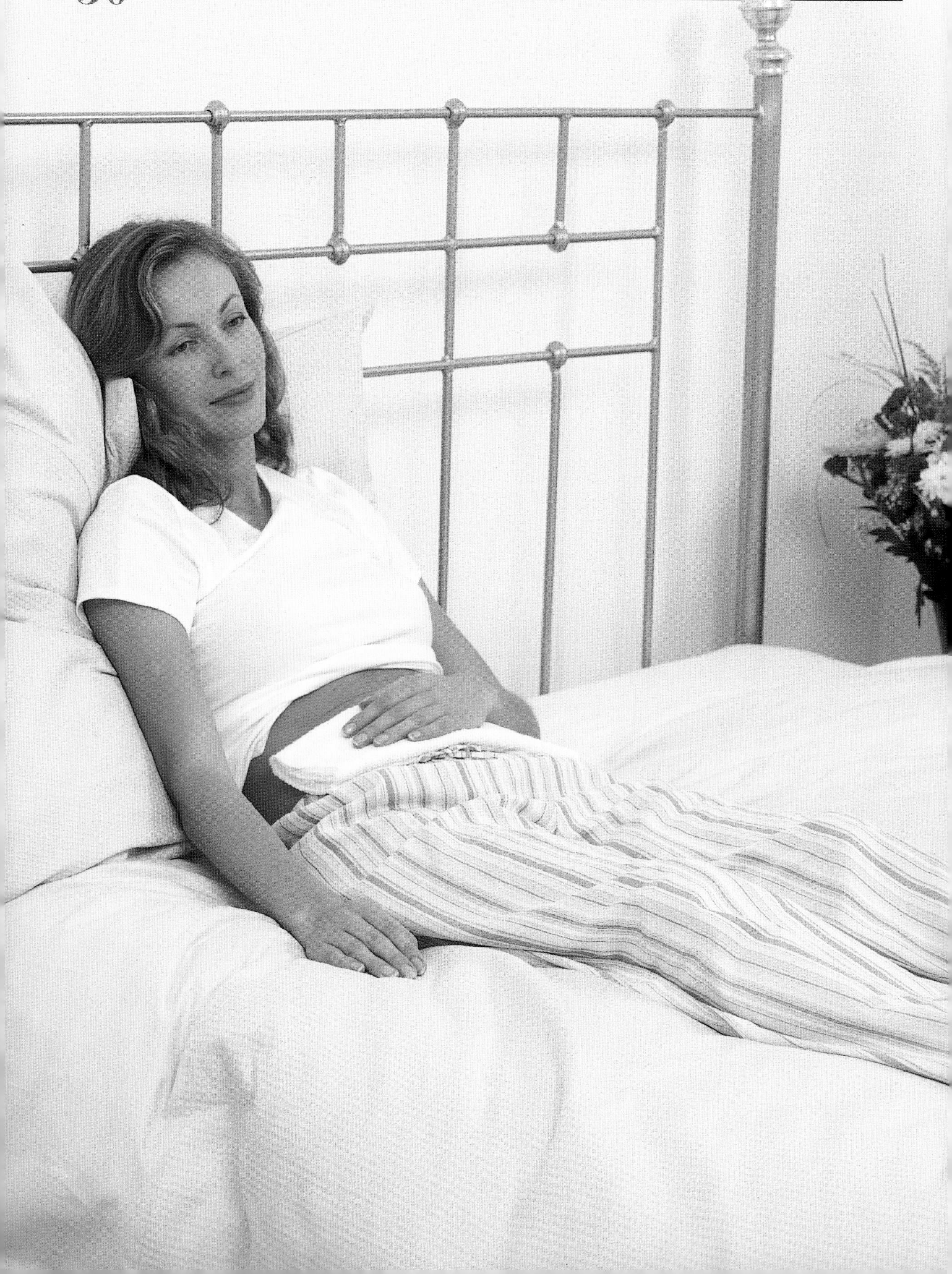

Ginger Compress

★ Take a dessertspoon of dried ginger or grate a 7–10-cm (3–4-inch) piece of fresh ginger.
★ Add it to a litre (1 ¾pt) of water and simmer this mixture slowly in a covered pan for 20 minutes to extract its therapeutic properties.
★ Allow the mix to cool enough so that it's hot, but not scalding.
★ Dip a cloth into the brew – a piece of small towelling is ideal because it is dense enough to hold the heat.
★ Wring the cloth out thoroughly and apply to the Tan Tien (see p. 29). The compress should feel hot, but not burning.
★ As the cloth cools, dip it into the ginger water

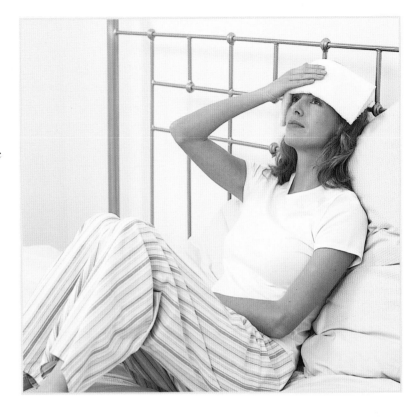

again. Keep repeating this until the water is too cool to be effective (after about 5 minutes). The ginger water can be kept refrigerated and reused several times, reheating it until it is hot to the touch each time.

Chamomile-lavender Compress

★ Take a tablespoon of dried chamomile and the same amount of lavender, or about a handful of each of the fresh herbs.
★ Add it to about half a litre (1¾pt) of boiling water, and allow it to infuse for 5 minutes.
★ Wring out a piece of cloth in the herbal mixture – a flannel (washcloth) is fine – and apply. The compress should feel hot,

but not scalding.
★ Relax – either sitting in a comfortable chair or lying down – and apply the hot compress to your brow for maximum effect. Breathe deeply, inhaling the soothing aroma and allowing the comforting warmth of the compress to help you let go of the mental clutter that so often prevents you from falling into a restful sleep.

An effective compress can also be made by using either of these herbs singly, or indeed by using them cold. In the latter case, simply allow the herbal mix to steep, strain it, allow it to cool, and refrigerate before use.

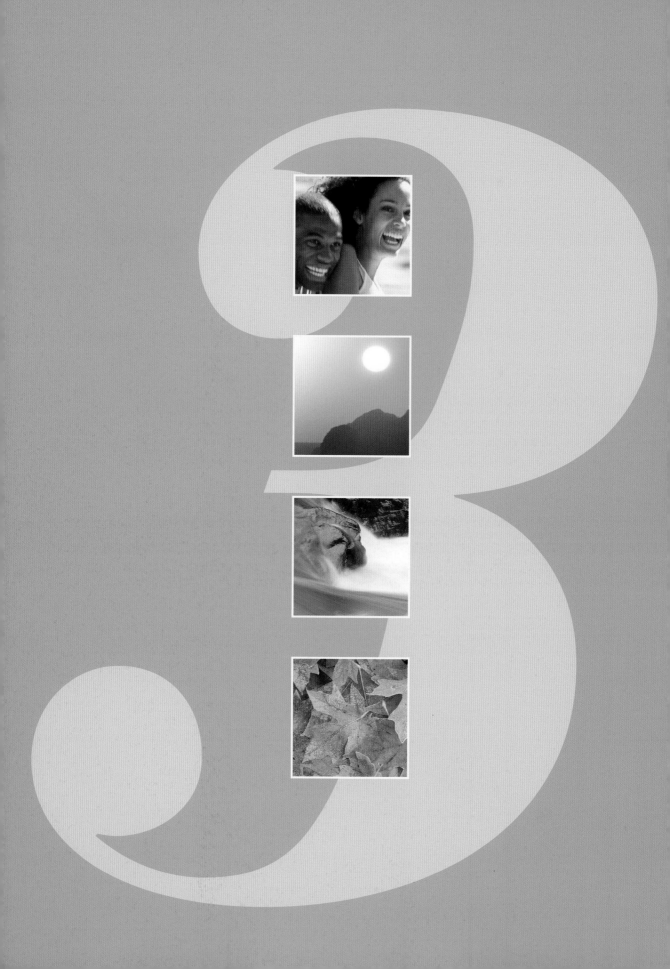

Chapter Three

ENERGY
Balancing

*Positive energy follows positive intent
and leads to peaceful sleep*

Exploring your energy field

Energy healing is an art that has been practised since time immemorial. It was, for a while, discounted in our modern, scientific society, but an awareness of its value, alongside (and complementing) more technological methods, is now emerging. It is safe and accessible, based in the knowledge that we are a complex network of interconnected energies – physically, mentally, emotionally, and spiritually.

Although we are very aware of our physical bodies, the less visible aspect of ourselves, the energy body (also known as the aura, or energy field), is often disregarded. This aspect of ourselves is, however, of great importance in terms of our overall health, because it acts as an invisible information highway, constantly giving and receiving messages to and from the environment around us. For example, we often have a hunch or gut feeling, which is a signal from our energy field – often about something or some-one in our vicinity. Emotions are also transmitted by means of our energy field. This means that by taking steps to heal our emotions, we can have a positive

HAPPY AND HEALTHY
When your life force, or chi, is balanced and flowing harmoniously, everything in life will seem easy, and you are likely to feel happy, healthy, and brimming with energy.

impact on our physical health. And, conversely, by improving the physical health of our bodies, we can have a positive effect on our emotional state.

For the purposes of this book we are concerned primarily with the meridian system (see p. 39), meridians being pathways that carry energy through the body. Traditional Chinese philosophy bases its healing methods – whether herbal, breath-related, diet-focused, massage-led or any other holistic approach – on ensuring that these pathways are kept clear and that the energy is flowing at a constant rate on all levels of being – physical, mental, emotional, and spiritual.

Balanced energy

When our energies are free-flowing and harmonious, we experience health and vitality on all levels of our being and life is a breeze in every way. We are equipped with all we need to meet and enjoy life to the full, welcoming challenges as a means of growth, learning, and expansion – and sleeping easily.

Imbalanced energy

However, when energies are failing to flow to their optimum, disruptions often occur. These are experienced as illness and problems such as an ability to switch off and get good-quality sleep. Blockages that occur in the energetic routes can, at the very least, produce feelings of being under the weather or a

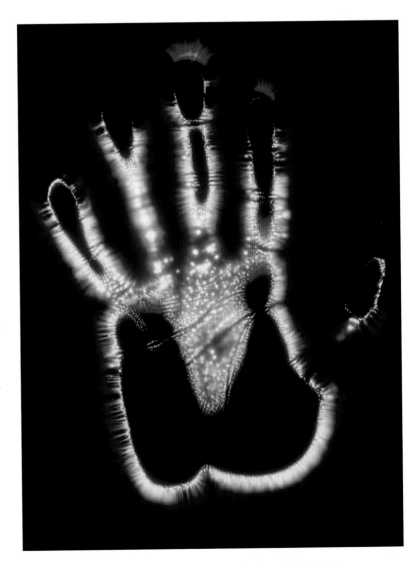

inability to "fire on all cylinders". And when these blockages become severe, then illness and exhaustion result.

ENERGETIC FIELD
The coloured areas in this kirlian photograph of a human hand are its electromagnetic discharges. Their shape, colour and form represent the aura of the hand.

The wise know that the way to health is balance; they are not overly concerned with worldly cares, but take time to look within, for therein lie the answers

Tuning into your energy

Whether we realize it or not, we are all aware of, and sensitive to, the energies within and around us. We can all feel the atmosphere in a room, we can tell, without speaking to someone, what sort of mood they are in. We know only too well when someone is angry or hostile toward us. We can sense, too, when someone has generous and loving feelings toward us.

We also know instinctively if we like someone or not as soon as we meet them – whether or not we are in tune with them. This is the silent language of energy.

Although we all have a certain awareness of this language, we can, of course, learn to become more aware of it (see exercise right) and proficient at it. This will allow us to have a greater understanding of ways in which we can improve not only our own health and vitality, but also those of our friends and family.

The healer within
Instances of us being in tune with other people's energy and thus making use of our "healer within" occur all the time – even though we might not know it. How often, for example, do we stroke a child's head when they are having trouble getting off to sleep? We are instinctively using a loving action to calm the mind and release tension, which, in turn, helps to bring about sleep. We also do things like rest our forehead in our hands or rub our forehead or temples when we need to clear our minds. So you see, a healing energy already lives within you. It's now just a matter of recognizing it, embracing it, and coaxing it out.

Sensing your energy
It is possible to experience the effects of your own energy flow (see exercise). With practice, you

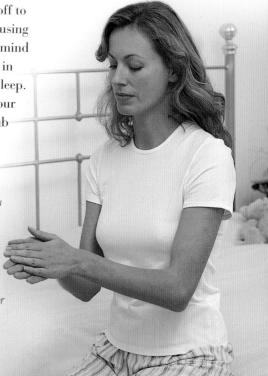

PALM RUBBING
The following exercise will allow you to try to tune into your own energy flow at any given moment. As with all exercises, or contemplations, the experience will become stronger with practice.

1 *Sit or stand in a relaxed manner and rub your palms briskly together for a moment or two.*

you will become more familiar with the language of energy and notice your own fluctuations. At times of stress and disturbed sleep, you will notice that your energy tends to be weak. When you have been well nourished by sleep, on the other hand, your energy will be flowing more strongly and you will have a greater resilience on all levels, being able to think more clearly and rise to all that life throws at you much more easily.

Professional healers

Many people in the healing profession have a natural gift for working positively with energies, but it is possible to acquire this skill through training and development. Energy healers, such as reiki practitioners and aromatherapists, are usually so in tune with the energies around them that they are able to "see" and "read" a person's energetic imbalances when treating them. Through the information

received via their aura, a healer is able to suggest, and perhaps introduce, some of the energetic changes needed to bring about a state of renewed balance and restored peace. Different healers use different techniques, whether reiki, herbalism, massage, acupuncture, aromatherapy, or any other form of treatment. These depend on their own individual preferences, as well as the preferences and needs of each person being treated.

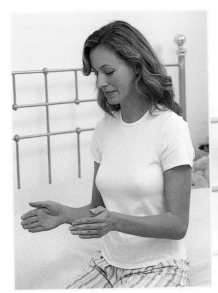

2 *Slowly separate your hands to a distance of about 15cm (6in), and focus on the space between your palms. Notice any sensations, such as warmth, tingling, or coolness.*

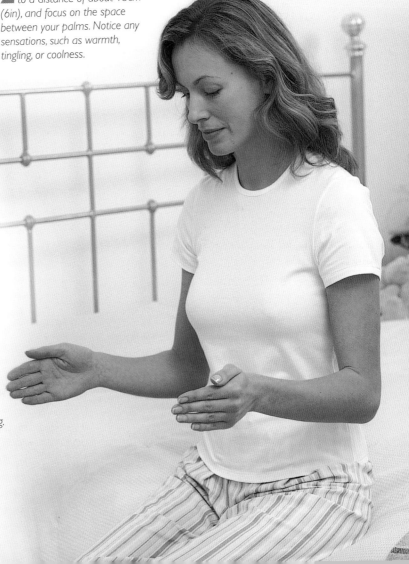

3 *Still focusing on this space, slowly separate your hands a little further. You may notice a stronger feeling between your palms, almost as though you are holding something. Gently move your hands toward each other very slightly, and then away. Do this several times, as though you are coaxing or forming something.*

Separate your hands a little further, still trying to maintain energetic contact between your palms. You may notice an increasing feeling of resistance.

Bring your hands slowly together again and notice the sensations between your palms.

The cycles *of* nature

Whether or not we are aware of it, we are influenced on a daily basis by the cycles of nature going on around us, as they create patterns of energy in our environment, which, in turn, affect our personal energy systems, and therefore our health.

The cycles of which we are most obviously aware are those of day and night, the months (the twenty-eight-day cycle of the moon), and the turning of the seasons. These cycles give a kind of coherence to life – indicating where we are at any given time and providing a natural and rhythmical structure to our lives. Indeed, they provide the foundations upon which we exist, measuring our time by the passage of light and darkness, and the rotations of the earth, moon, and sun.

Daily peaks and dips
Traditional Chinese philosophy teaches us that during the 24-hour cycle of one day and night, our natural energy flows through one full cycle – peaking and dipping through each of our major energy systems. Because there are twelve major systems – each one relating to an organ or physical part of the body (see right) – each one peaks or dips for a two-hour period in a natural sequence (see pp. 40–41). This means that for a two-hour period out of twenty-four, one particular function is at its highest and most active, able to take in and absorb natural energy. Twelve hours later, this same function is at its lowest, which could be thought of as the function's "resting" time. We often have an instinctive awareness of this energetic flow, noticing that we are

Main Meridian Functions

Large intestine: *awakens the ability to condense and simplify things*
Stomach: *encourages self-nourishment and appreciation of all that is good*
Spleen: *provides the ability to transform and move on*
Heart: *stirs feelings of love and compassion*
Small intestine: *helps us make sound judgements*
Bladder: *encourages us to seek out balance in our lives*
Gall bladder: *encourages us to put plans and ideas into action*
Liver: *brings vitality, growth, and creativity*
Kidney: *gives us the strength and fluidity to welcome change*
Lung: *gives the ability to receive from the present and release from the past*
Circulation-sex: *regulates circulation and hormonal function*
Triple warmer: *regulates heat and fluid in the body*

habitually tired, moody, alert, or creative at specific times.

Meridian system

It is also thought that there are twelve major invisible pathways through the body, each one servicing a particular organ or function (see box right). These are called "meridians" and form an energetic network that affects every process in the body, including the endocrine, digestive, respiratory, musculo-skeletal, and nervous systems. Each process is supplied with energy by at least one meridian, and if the energy supply is good, the health of that particular process will also be good. When this network is fully functioning, and all systems are working in harmony, all is therefore well and quality sleep should be a natural part of the body's cycle. However, there are many factors

that will disrupt the sensitive system, such as an inappropriate diet, emotional disturbances, and stress. The body is often able to rebalance itself, given the correct conditions, if the problems are only temporary. However, over a sustained period of time these disruptions can emerge as symptoms that disturb our quality of life on a more long-term basis, such as insomnia.

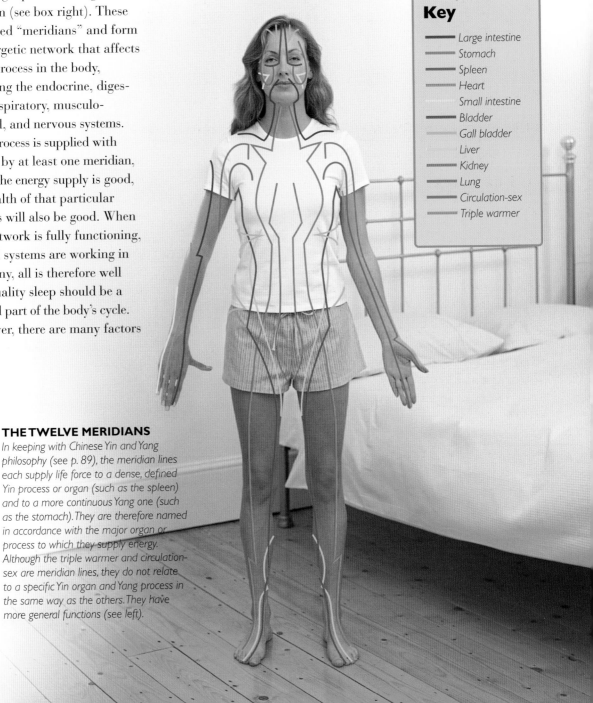

Key

▬▬▬	*Large intestine*
▬▬▬	*Stomach*
▬▬▬	*Spleen*
▬▬▬	*Heart*
▬▬▬	*Small intestine*
▬▬▬	*Bladder*
▬▬▬	*Gall bladder*
▬▬▬	*Liver*
▬▬▬	*Kidney*
▬▬▬	*Lung*
▬▬▬	*Circulation-sex*
▬▬▬	*Triple warmer*

THE TWELVE MERIDIANS

In keeping with Chinese Yin and Yang philosophy (see p. 89), the meridian lines each supply life force to a dense, defined Yin process or organ (such as the spleen) and to a more continuous Yang one (such as the stomach). They are therefore named in accordance with the major organ or process to which they supply energy. Although the triple warmer and circulation-sex are meridian lines, they do not relate to a specific Yin organ and Yang process in the same way as the others. They have more general functions (see left).

24-hour cycle

By developing an awareness that each of us is part of, and therefore subject to, natural forces, we can begin to understand the ebbs and flows of energy that we experience in a 24-hour cycle. We can then harness and learn from the lessons that these cycles bring.

By relating your own disturbed sleeping pattern to the time slots on the following pages, you are likely to gain valuable insights as to which potentially optimal body function might be imbalanced, and therefore be causing your insomnia.

Day & night: 11–1

Some people find it extremely hard to get off to sleep when they go to bed, but once asleep they manage to have a fairly restful time. This initial period may be quite distressing, because however tired you thought you were, as soon as you go to bed, you are suddenly wide awake. The time between 11 pm and 1 am is the potentially optimal time of the gall bladder, with a corresponding daytime energy of the heart system. Imbalances of these energies are common in people with stressful lifestyles. These people may have positions of responsibility from which they find it very hard to switch off. They may feel overly burdened and responsible and find it hard to make sound decisions. Life may feel rather joyless as work threatens to engulf all other pursuits.

Day & night: 1–3

A very common time for wakefulness is between 1 and 3 am, when the liver energy is at its highest. Liver energy relates to the storage of unresolved issues, involving anger and frustration. If you look at the corresponding time during the day, 1 to 3 pm, you will see that it is the time of the small intestine, which is the organ through which we are able to digest, both in terms of the physical digestion of food, and the mental and emotional digestion of problems. We can therefore develop a picture of a person with difficulties in sleeping at this time during the night as someone who finds it hard to resolve emotional conflict, particularly that which has provoked feelings of anger, frustration, or resentment.

Day & night: 3–5

Let us look at the period between 3 and 5 am, which is the time of highest lung energy. The corresponding daytime energy is the bladder system. The lungs are the means through which we experience grief, sadness, and depression – feelings of loss. Very often lung complaints, such as bronchitis, asthma, and pneumonia, are thought to be related to emotional loss or despair – feelings of not being able to breathe as you simply cannot take in enough air. The corresponding daytime energy of the bladder system is associated with the nervous system – this meridian runs the length of the spine. Imbalances in these energy systems cause someone to be sad, depressed, edgy, or nervy, and unable to fully relax and put events behind them. They may wake suddenly in the night: the mind unable to relax or close down, and the body restless, fidgety, and uncomfortable.

Day & night: 5–7

Some people find it fairly easy to get off to sleep and rest soundly all night, but waken too early in the morning – perhaps as the dawn chorus is beginning and the rest of the world still seems to be sleeping. This is the time between 5 and 7 am and is the energy peak of the large intestine, with a corresponding daytime energy of the kidney system. Wakefulness at this time – if it is causing disturbance – gives a picture of someone whose foundations are feeling a bit shaky. They are finding life somewhat daunting as they struggle to find their feet. They

may be timid and nervous and wake up with an empty, hollow feeling in the stomach. There are, however, many people who enjoy waking at this time, finding it a good opportunity to see to activities that benefit from quiet time and a clear mind.

Day & night: 7–9

Most of us do not go to bed this early in the evening, so are not concerned with this imbalance in relation to insomnia. However, this period is related to the energy system of the circulation, with a corresponding daytime energy of the stomach. An imbalance here leads to feeling stuck in your approach to life and worrying about prospective changes.

Day & night: 9–11

Although we might be ready for bed during this period in the evening, we are often not ready to go to sleep. This period is therefore not explored as a time of distress for people suffering from insomnia. It relates to the energy system called the

triple warmer (which regulates body heat), and the corresponding daytime energy of the spleen. Imbalance in these systems is indicated by a difficulty concentrating for long and a tendency to worry excessively. This imbalance can be prevalent at times when there are too many pressures or decisions to contend with, and life appears to be overwhelming. Spleen energy is also connected with the ability to resist harmful external influences, whether in terms of good immunity to illness, or simply not being too easily sucked in to other people's ideas, which may be at odds with your own.

A person's emotional state is as much an indication of energetic imbalance as their physical symptoms

Personal patterns

Many of us have a particular period during the day when we feel at our best. You may be a morning person, springing happily into action at the first hint of daylight, but finding that you run out of steam later on in the day. Or you may perhaps be a night-time person, coming to life as the rest of us are flagging – able to work or play through the evening, and sometimes deep into the night. Or you may, as many of us do, fall somewhere between these two. We are all responding to our natural rhythms and personal energy flows, and provided that you feel well and healthy and your life is not suffering from disruption, this is absolutely fine.

Applying this system

If you find, however, that you wake, annoyingly, at a certain time every night, you may be able to relate your pattern to the peak and trough time slots (see pp. 40–41). Perhaps you recognize some of the emotional symptoms and can relate them to your own life and feelings.

The ideal is for all the energy systems to flow together harmoniously, each one supporting the next, and although there can be numerous reasons for disruption of this ideal flow, the root of the problem often lies in our emotional life. You may have dismissed a thought or feeling as unimportant but, in fact, come to realize that it needs attention. This could, for example, be underlying feelings of anger or aggression, which cause disharmony in the energetic function of the liver; or feelings of timidity and fear, which

MORNING OR NIGHT-TIME?
Decide which kind of person you are and work on that aspect.

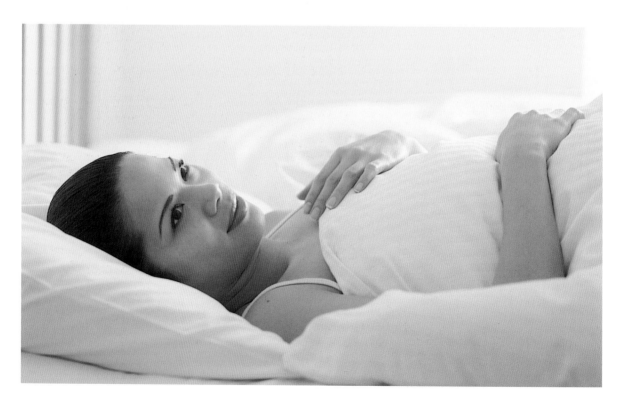

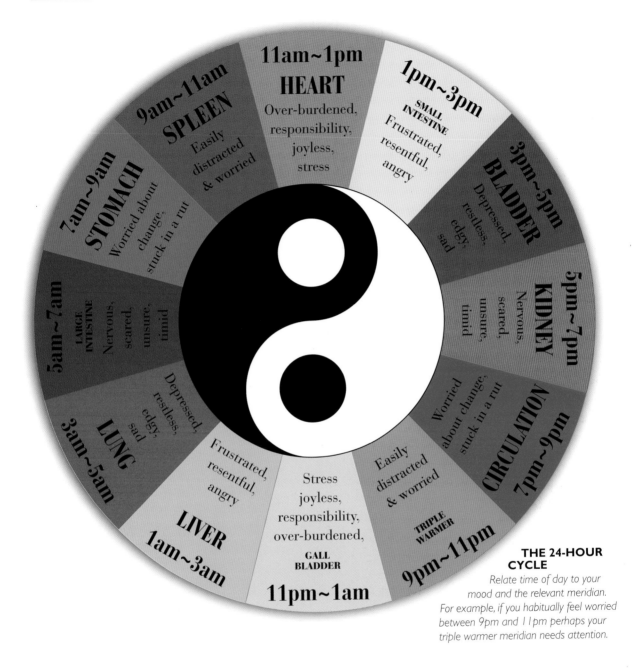

THE 24-HOUR CYCLE

Relate time of day to your mood and the relevant meridian. For example, if you habitually feel worried between 9pm and 11pm perhaps your triple warmer meridian needs attention.

restrict your decision-making ability, causing imbalances in the kidney system, thus disrupting sleep. Even if they are long-buried feelings, they nevertheless have a bearing on the health and balance of your energetic stability. Or perhaps your periods of wakefulness span more than one of the time phases, and thus relate to a mixture of emotional disturbances. Whatever the cause, you will find a whole range of techniques and exercises within this book to help you realign any imbalances. The meridian massage techniques on pages 54–61 may be particularly helpful as they relate specifically to the time slots of sleeplessness explained here.

The diagram above gives a pictorial view of our energy flow over a 24-hour period. The organ mentioned is the one that is at its potential peak at that time.

5 seasons, 5 elements

There are many natural cycles that have a great impact on our lives and provide us with important reference points, but one of the most significant ones is the wondrous, beautiful changing of the seasons throughout the course of each year.

In traditional Chinese philosophy, the five seasons of the Chinese year are thought to correspond not only to the five elements, but also to the five major organs in the body and what are believed to be the primary emotions (see right). These seasons – a source of external life force – affect us

just as much as the meridian systems within us. The seasons include an additional Indian summer, or harvest time, which is set apart from summer and autumn in the Chinese calendar.

If we take the year as a whole, we will see that each season and element takes its natural place,

flowing from the previous one and into the next. The idea of perfect balance is to include all of these aspects in our personalities – but very often one or two predominate.

Putting it into action

Although we often have the tendency to follow the overriding emotion of whatever season it is, being more inclined to introspection in the winter, more cheery and active in the spring, happier in the summer sun, more mellow and contented at harvest time, and going into a more reflective state again in the autumn, this is

The wise man watches the flow of the river

He watches the turning of the seasons

He watches the stirrings in the heavens

And knows that he, too, must be guided by

His own seasons, his own stirrings, and his own flow

For this is "The Way"

THE FIVE ELEMENTS

This chart illustrates how closely linked seasonal and "elemental" imbalances are to extreme emotional states (see also pp. 46–49).

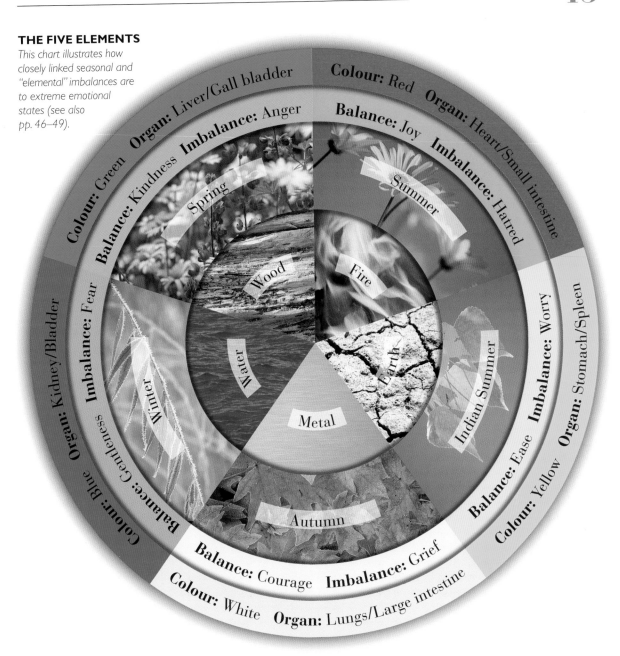

by no means the whole picture. We can, of course, experience any kind of emotion at any time, but by achieving an understanding of the cycle of the five seasons and their connections with our physical and emotional qualities, we can have more choice over how we proceed. For example, you may

be feeling weepy and exhausted, beset by problem after problem, unable to sleep and recuperate. Tears seem to flow at every opportunity. If you apply the guidelines of the five seasons, you will notice that you have hit a "winter" phase: an imbalance in the kidney and bladder meridians, which is likely to

correspond to the water element – hence the weepiness. You can then know and gain comfort from the fact that what you are experiencing is an indication of an energetic and "elemental" imbalance, and can take steps, using the suggestions offered in this book as your guide, to bring yourself back to harmony again.

Spring

Spring is the wood element, which is related to fresh new ideas and vigorous growth as the days become longer. The image associated with wood is that of coming deep from the earth – with strong, flexible roots – yet rising confidently toward the skies. We feel this vitality echoed in our tendency to want to make plans and revive our dreams at this time of joy and rebirth – now that the quiet introspection of winter is at an end.

The colour is a bright, clear green and its corresponding organs and energy systems are the liver and gall bladder. It is said that when these systems are in perfect balance and at optimum flow, the emotional quality expressed will be that of progressing through life with kindness to all beings. Someone dominated by the wood element will display great strength and endurance and will be capable of making clear and informed decisions – aiming to reach even higher, like the branches of a tree. When this system is out of balance and ambitions thwarted, however, it can quickly lead to anger, irritability, muddled thinking, and frustration. This can, in turn, lead to headaches and sleeplessness. The eyes are also governed by the wood element, making it essential we keep it in balance to maintain clear-sightedness.

Hear the wisdom in the simplicity of Mother Nature's dance; let your spirit lift and soar, filled with the spark of fresh morning green

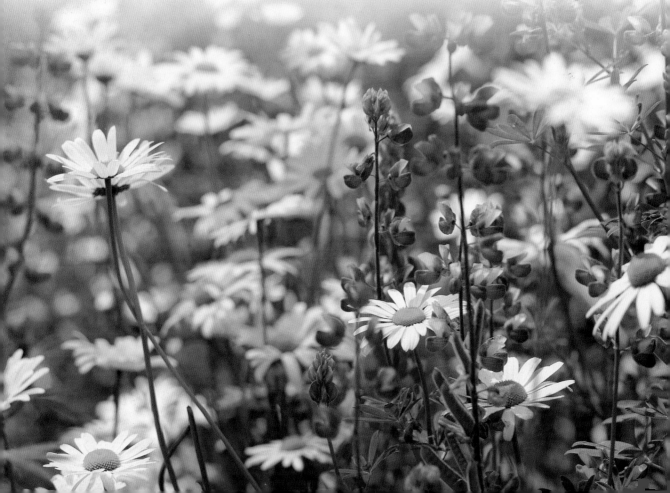

Summer

Summer is the element of fire, bringing heat, excitement, love, joy, and action to our lives. This is the time of the highest activity and the most light – the time for sharing and creating warmth and laughter in relationships with people close to you.

Bright red symbolizes the fire element. The heart and small intestine are the organs and energy systems that are relevant, and when these are in perfect balance, life is full and over-flowing with joy and laughter. Summer people tend to live through the forces of their hearts – being loving, exuberant, and energetic. When out of balance, however, jealousies and mean-ness can emerge. It becomes hard to feel good about oneself or other people, and choices and decisions become increasingly difficult to make. It feels as though disharmony reigns over your life. This imbalance is often the one experienced by workaholics and is the one most commonly responsible for disturbances in sleep patterns – an excess of fire makes it hard to cool off and for sleep to come.

Indian summer

Indian summer is the time of the earth element, when we can feast on the abundance of Mother Nature, nurturing and nourishing ourselves on the deepest levels. This is the time for gathering together and creating a strong centre, from which all else can flow. The organs and systems relating to the earth element are the stomach and spleen, and the colour is the glorious yellow of a full sun. When this element is in balance, the voice takes on a musical quality – singing the richness of life. But when there is disharmony in these energy systems, there is a tendency to overthink, make unnecessary complications for yourself, and possibly mistrust our own judge-ment. Life becomes a worry, resulting in fatigue and poor sleeping habits.

Let sun and joy banish all cares, for they are as passing shadows in the face of the mighty sun

Autumn

Autumn is related to the metal element and is the time for delving deep within ourselves to find strength and courage. It is the time for thinking back over the past, telling old stories, and bringing to the surface feelings that have been buried; for gathering together the harvest of our learning, sharing our knowledge, and reflecting on the future – perhaps gaining insight as to how we can break our pattern of disturbed sleep.

The colour is white, and the organs and energy systems are the lungs and large intestine, as well as the skin and hair. When these are well balanced, emotional

Stand in the golden valley and on the misty hillside, gaze upon all that is, know that each cry of pain and each shout of laughter has brought you to this moment – and all is well

strength is at its peak, equipping us to face even the most difficult of life's challenges, such as bereavements, with honesty. We allow ourselves to feel the emotions, and then to let them go when the time has passed.

When imbalance occurs, on the other hand, sadness and grief become locked away, which can lead to a lack of energy flow to the whole body, as it struggles to breathe in sufficient energy, making restful sleep a problem.

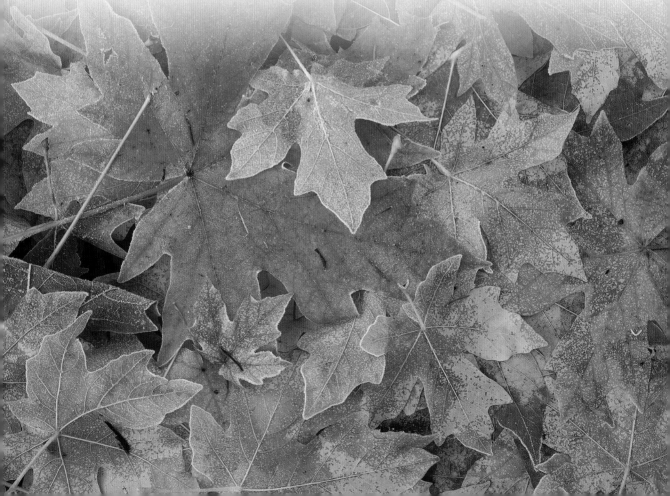

Winter

Lastly, we continue into winter and the water element, which is so variable and ever-changing – moving from the gentlest trickling brook to the deepest, calmest of lakes, to the mighty ocean, and even to the complete stillness of frozen ice. This element, when in balance, mirrors our variable natures and our infinite flexibility. This is the element of the kidney and bladder energies, which is represented by the colour blue. We are encouraged by the stillness of the season to look calmly within, using the different faces of the water element as our guide. When out of harmony, however, this inner journeying can be experienced as the inability to control irrational fears – a feeling of being bombarded by all the seemingly meaningless things that life throws at our feet. This could be thought of as the inability to be still or fluid for long enough to look within and can lead to chronic anxiety, which is depleting to the whole body. Disruption in this energy system causes a general feeling of overload and of being burnt out – making sleep seem almost impossible and allowing exhaustion to set in.

Listen to the quiet words as they arise from the frozen stillness, seek only the pure, and the impure will be washed away by the waters of life

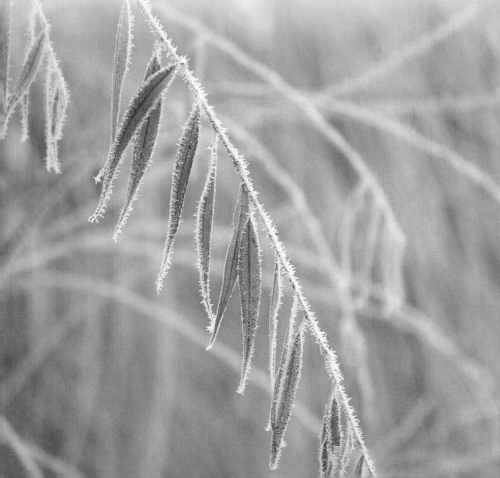

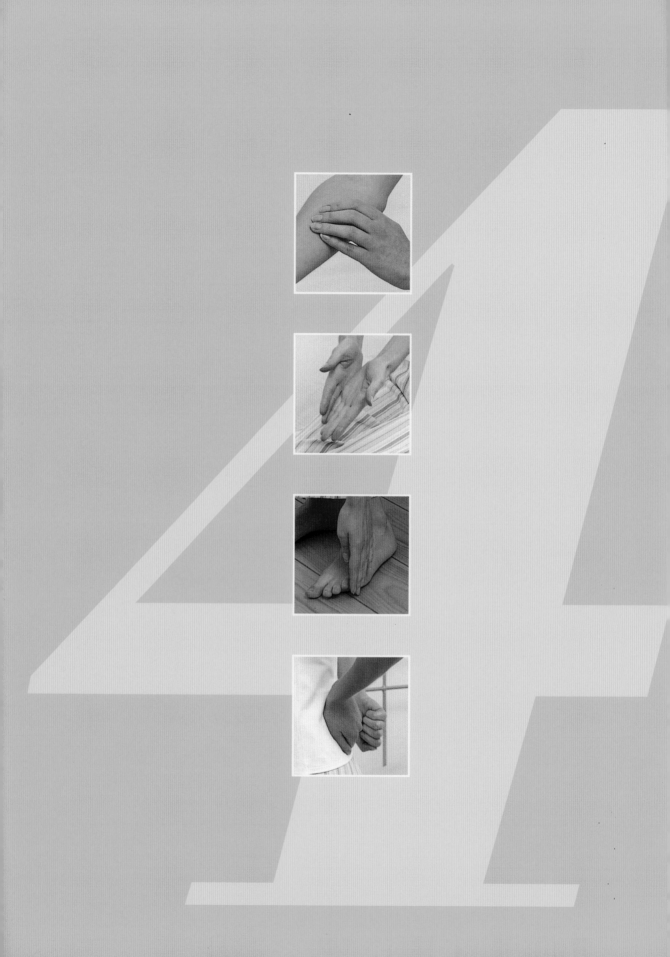

Chapter Four

MASSAGING

your meridians

Activate the chi –
the breath of life,
the energy of existence,
the spark that ignites

The healing touch

The following Chinese meridian massage techniques are designed to work on the energy lines of your own body, flushing out old energy and introducing new energy, in order to help remove blockages and create the balance required for restful sleep and recuperation. They are simple to perform and take precious little time to do, yet can bring great rewards.

The more time you take, the deeper your concentration, and the more positive your intent when you do the self-massages on the following pages, the greater and swifter their effects will be.

Try to spend at least ten minutes – morning and evening (or when awake during the night) – doing the one (or several) most relevant to you to promote a healthy flow of energy. They are split down into time slots throughout the night (based on Oriental thinking; see pp. 40–41) so that you can choose those that best suit your needs.

Alternatively, if you have a friend or partner who is willing to help you, they could try out the techniques on your body for you. And remember that drinking some water will enhance the effects.

What to do

It is generally recommended to drink at least a litre (2 pints) of fresh water a day, but always have a drink of water before beginning to massage too. Then wash and dry your hands, and vigorously shake them and rub them together until they feel warm and alive. Either sit, lie, or stand, depending on which of your meridians you plan to work on, but make sure that you can relax thoroughly in order to encourage you to work slowly and deliberately. You can either massage directly onto the skin, or through clothing; it is just as effective either way. Use either your palms or

STAY HYDRATED
It's always important to drink plenty of fresh water, but it is particularly crucial when doing any of the exercises in this book as all energy work is more effective when the body is hydrated.

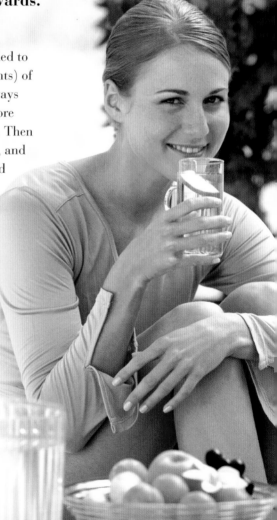

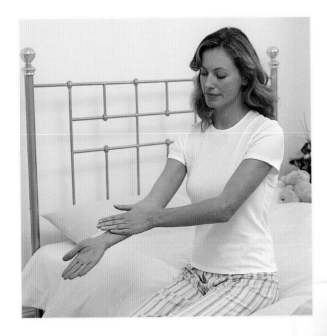

MERIDIAN MASSAGE
You can choose to work with either one hand or both when massaging the meridians, and with either the fingertips or the palms of the hands – whichever you feel more comfortable doing, as the most important thing is positive, relaxed intention.

fingers to trace a line along the section of the meridian lines indicated – instructions on how to do each one are given on the following pages. You can work with one hand or both, depending on which comes more easily to you, and you can start on either side of the body. The main thing is to feel at ease and relaxed, so that your energy is focused on the positive intention behind the massage, rather than the massage technique. A calm and focused mind has the power

and potential to move energy. You may feel a warmth or tingling when performing these massages, which is a sign that you are effecting positive changes.

The feeling that you want to achieve is that of flushing out the old and sweeping in the new. You therefore direct the energy first one way in order to cleanse, and then the other in order to encourage renewed flow. In general, we use three sweeps to free up blockages, followed by

six to encourage full flow in the right direction. Good breathing (see pp. 74–75) is important as it encourages a healthy flow of energy. Try to time each sweep along the meridian with one full out-breath to enhance the flow of the energy. And use each deep, abdominal inward breath to balance and restore you between energy sweeps. Take a few moments after completing each sequence to relax and appreciate any changes in your energy flow.

Difficulty in *falling asleep:*

11pm–1am

There are many times when it can be difficult to fall asleep when you first go to bed, however tired or exhausted you feel at the end of a long and demanding day. As soon as your head hits the pillow, as if by magic, you are wide awake.

This indicates that there are imbalances in your gall bladder meridian (wood element) and your heart meridian (fire element). The fire has become too strong in the body and is consuming the wood to your detriment. It must therefore be calmed down, and the wood element stimulated.

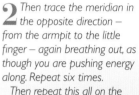

2 *Then trace the meridian in the opposite direction – from the armpit to the little finger – again breathing out, as though you are pushing energy along. Repeat six times.*
Then repeat this all on the other arm.

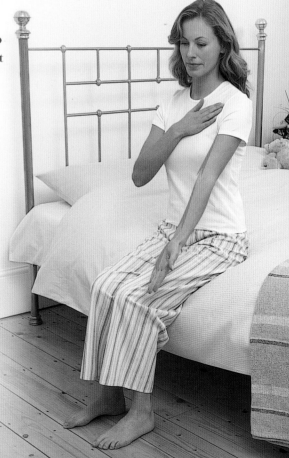

CALMING THE FIRE: HEART MERIDIAN
This is to bring coolness and harmony, releasing latent feelings of tightness engrained in your outlook on life.

1 *Outstretch your arm, palm facing up, and, with your other hand, start tracing a line from the outside edge of the little finger, up the inside of the arm, to the armpit area. Repeat three times. Breathe out each time you trace the line, and use the inward breaths to restore you between sweeps.*

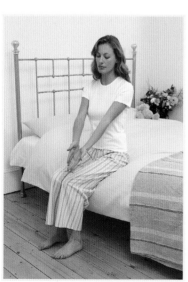

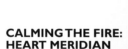

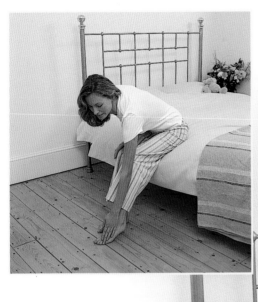

INVIGORATING THE WOOD: GALL BLADDER MERIDIAN

This helps to restore feelings of gentleness: everything will return to how it should be, with its own place and its own timing.

1 *Starting at the outside edge of the fourth toe, trace a line up the outside of the leg, to the waist. Repeat three times, breathing out as you draw up, and using the inward breaths to balance and restore you between sweeps.*

2 *Reverse the direction, again breathing out as you push the energy along. Repeat six times.*
Then repeat it all on the other leg.

HEART   **GALL BLADDER**

1am–3am
Sleeplessness

There are nights when you no sooner seem to have fallen off into an exhausted and much-needed sleep, when, there you are, wide awake again – the thought of returning to the peaceful world of dreams now seeming like a far-off impossibility.

This indicates imbalances in the liver (wood element) and the small intestine (fire element) – the same elements as in the previous phase of sleeplessness.

An excess of "fire" in the energy systems of the body is, in fact, one of the most common causes of sleeplessness. This is often because we don't take enough time to release daily stresses and tensions, allowing them to rear up at those very times when we most need rest.

2 *Reverse the direction, beginning at the edge of the little finger and tracing a line up to the back of the shoulder. Once again, breathe out as you do it to push the energy along. Repeat six times.*
Then repeat the whole process on the other arm.

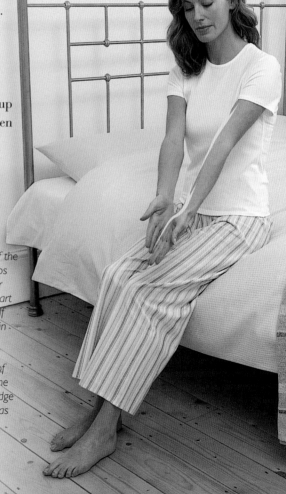

CALMING THE FIRE: SMALL INTESTINE MERIDIAN

At times like these, concerns of the heart frequently arise – perhaps concerns about relationships or family members. Calm your heart and mind, by reminding yourself that these are best dealt with in daylight hours.

1 *Reach to the centre back of the shoulder and trace a line from here down to the outer edge of the little finger. Breathe out as you do this to draw the energy along. Repeat three times.*

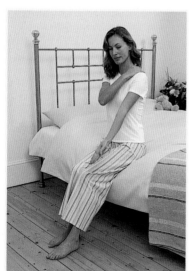

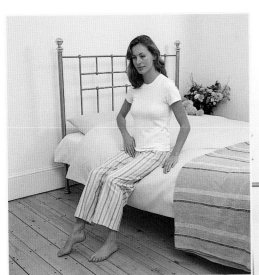

INVIGORATING THE WOOD: LIVER MERIDIAN

It is crucial to allow frustrations to disperse in the knowledge that frustration can stop progress. An attitude of gentleness is one from which solutions can arise.

1 *Starting in the groin, trace a line down the inside of the leg, to the outside edge of the big toe, breathing out as you draw the energy along the meridian. Repeat three times.*

2 *Reverse the direction, starting with the outside edge of the big toe, and finishing in the groin. Again, breathe out as you massage in order to push the energy along. Repeat six times.*
   Then repeat all this on the other leg.

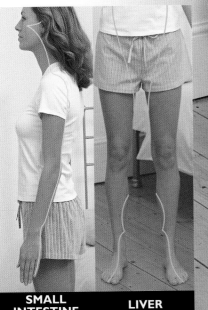

SMALL INTESTINE   **LIVER**

3am–5am
Sleeplessness

At times, you may snap awake between 3 and 5 in the morning, feeling as if you're being dragged slowly awake by an effort of some unseen force. You lie awake tossing and turning, unable to find ease or comfort as fears and worries race around your head.

2 *Reverse the direction, starting wherever you stopped step 1, and draw a line down to the outer edge of the foot. Breathe out, as though pushing energy along. Repeat six times.*
Then repeat the whole process on the other side of the body.

This indicates imbalances in the lungs (metal element) and the bladder (water element). The water has become torrential, threatening to wash away the metal, and must be brought back into balance. Be honest with yourself and wise enough to recognize the difference between the irrational fears that may seem ridiculous in the light of day and the concerns that you have brushed aside or put to the back of your mind, but which will need addressing sooner or later.

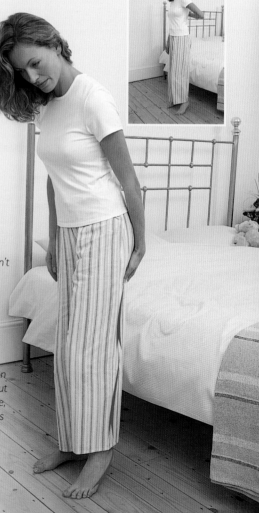

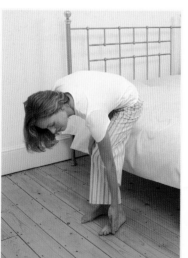

CALMING THE STORM: BLADDER MERIDIAN
It is useful to utter words of comfort to yourself while doing this massage. "Don't worry" and "It's alright" are helpful.

1 *Starting at the outside edge of the little toe, trace a line along the outside of the foot to the ankle. Move your hand up behind the ankle, to the centre of the calf, and up your thigh to the centre of the buttock. Then reach on up the spine, as high as you can without strain. If this last stage is uncomfortable, simply stop at the thigh. Breathe out as you draw energy along this meridian. Repeat three times.*

STRENGTHENING THE METAL: LUNG MERIDIAN

Try to allay your fears while doing this massage with affirmations of resolve and courage, such as "I will address the situations that need attention, but in the right way and at the right time."

1 Starting at the outer edge of the thumb, trace a line up the inside of the arm, over the front of the shoulder, onto the upper ribs and ending toward the centre of the chest, in a natural line with the arm. Breathe out as you do this to draw the energy along. Repeat three times.

2 Reverse the direction by beginning with the hand in the centre of the chest — at the approximate position of the lung. Trace a line down the inside of the arm to the thumb. Breathe out as you massage to encourage the energy to be pushed along the meridian. Repeat six times.

Then repeat all this on the other side.

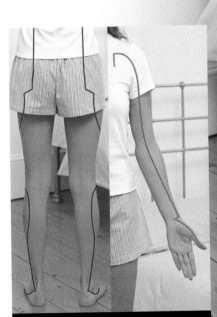

BLADDER   **LUNG**

Wakefulness 5am–7am

Often it might feel as though the whole world is wrapped in peaceful slumber when you are wide awake at this early hour, without any desire to be. Exhaustion and despair after yet another insufficient night's sleep may well start to set in.

2 *Reverse the direction, starting with the point underneath the foot, and ending at the inner thigh. Again, breathe out as you massage to push energy along. Repeat six times.*
Then repeat both steps on the other leg.

If you wake at this time and do not feel that you have had sufficient sleep, or if you are unlucky enough still not to have fallen asleep, the indications are of an imbalance in the large intestine (metal element) and the kidneys (water element). The water is flowing too rapidly to bring about a state of rest. We need to aim to achieve a gently meandering river, moving around the landscape, rather than ploughing destructively through everything in its path – including the metal.

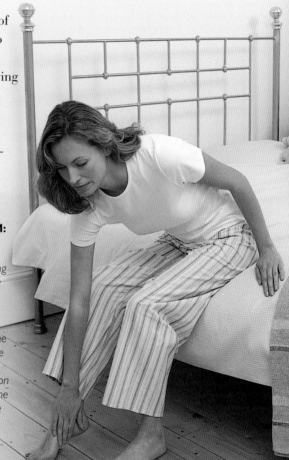

CALMING THE STORM: KIDNEY MERIDIAN

This is a time to be kind to yourself, knowing and accepting that you will work through any difficult emotions in your own time.

1 *Starting on the inside of the thigh, trace a line down the inside of the leg, down to the instep, and ending on a point on the ball of the foot, between the second and third toes. Breathe out as you do this to draw energy along this line. Repeat three times.*

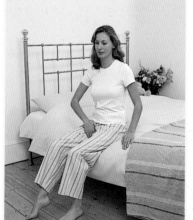

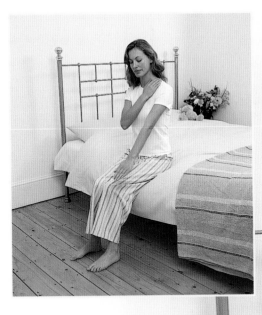

STRENGTHENING THE METAL: LARGE INTESTINE

Use this massage time to remind yourself that you have the inner resources to cope with whatever comes your way.

1 Start at the top of the shoulder, close to the neck, and trace a line straight down to the outside edge of the index finger. Breathe out as you do this to draw energy along this line. Repeat three times.

2 Reverse the direction, starting at the outside edge of the index finger, and ending on top of the shoulder. Breathe out as you massage to push the energy along. Repeat six times.
   Then repeat the whole massage process on the other arm.

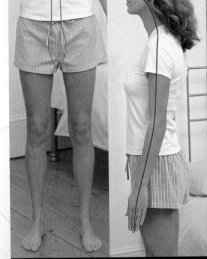

LARGE INTESTINE   **KIDNEY**

Instant stress-release *points*

The more relaxed our minds and bodies are, the better our energy will flow. The better our energy flows, the more our health will improve. And the healthier we are, the better we will tend to sleep at night. So how can we learn to relax at the drop of a hat?

The mind has a great influence over the energetic body. This is because the energetic bodies are made up of those invisible parts of us that are, nevertheless, very real – such as our thoughts, emotions, and feelings. Because the mind plays a very significant part in the health of our energy body, it can either work for us, helping to balance the energy flow and bringing about good health, or it can work against us, causing disruptions and diminishing our overall health. Conditions such as insomnia indicate that the body is struggling and that there are energetic imbalances, which will require time and effort to put right.

One way of getting yourself back on the road to recovery is to focus on two very effective stress-release points, or holding points, on your forehead about 2½ cm (1 in) up from the centre of your eyebrows (see right). We quite often naturally place our hands here when feeling stressed or anxious, but it is useful to do it consciously and to direct your energy here when your mind refuses to quieten down, or when you are unable to sleep, despite both your mind and your body being exhausted.

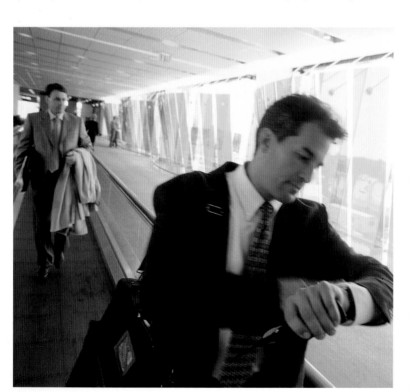

STRESSFUL TIMES
Holding the stress-release points on your forehead during times of high stress could prevent you from feeling quite so pressurized when things aren't going your way.

EMOTIONAL RELEASE

The same stress-release points are helpful in releasing the emotions related to a traumatic event, such as a bereavement or break-up, which is keeping you awake at night. Although it is impossible to change the event – and highly unhealthy to bury traumas or pretend they didn't happen – we can, nevertheless, change the emotions associated with them. Although the technique can be practised on oneself, it is even more effective if a sympathetic friend or relative does it on you. It can be done at any time of the day.

★ *Either stand behind the recipient and place one finger from each of your hands on the stress-relief points, or stand to the side of them, placing the thumb and middle finger of one hand on the pressure points and using the other hand to support the back of their head. Then concentrate on beaming clear, calming energy toward them. The recipient should then relive the traumatic event disturbing them in their mind's eye. Do not try to influence the person. Simply give them the help they need to free themselves. Stay calm and gentle if any difficult feelings come to the surface, knowing that they will soon pass, leaving a sense of relief.*

Author's Advice

When I used these quick and simple techniques to help my daughter, it had such a profound effect on her that she said she felt as though negative energy actually left her body there and then. The healing effects were immediate.

INCREASED CLARITY

Holding your stress-release points for a minute or two can bring tremendous relief from the turmoils of the mind. Use them whenever tensions are building, when you feel the need for increased clarity, or when you think your inability to sleep is due to stress and anxiety.

★ *Gently place your thumb and index or middle finger in position to induce calm. After a while you will probably notice that your breathing deepens and flows more freely and that your mind is clearer. You should also find that you have more control over your thoughts and sleep becomes more possible. In fact, you may even have some interesting insights as your thoughts become less congested.*

Release *the* fear

It's really easy to feel almost paralyzed by fear when life seems to throw endless streams of challenges our way. However, by remembering to turn inward to the stillness at our core, we can find what we need to deal with situations, as they arise.

If we are prepared to tune in and listen to our bodies and take note of fluctuations in our energy, we can use the knowledge gained as our personal guide. Have you noticed, for example, that, if you are doing something you really enjoy, time flies, you feel highly energized, and life feels good? If, however, you are trying to do something for which you have no desire, you may feel tired, irritable, or impatient. The latter are the sort of tasks you should try to let go of in order to free up your time and energy. Sometimes, just shedding certain burdens from your life is enough to bring about balance, renewed health, and quality sleep.

It can, however, prove very difficult to let go of situations, or people who have been a big part of your life. We have the tendency to hold on to that with which we are familiar and fear that which is unfamiliar – even if it is the unfamiliarity of having more time on our hands. It can therefore be terrifying to contemplate the release of the known routine and to begin an exploration into change.

Fear-related insomnia

Insomnia can be symptomatic of this fear – the inability to let go enough to allow your body to sleep. We fear that our world will fall apart if we aren't in control 24 hours a day. And we love to hang on to it so much that sleep seems like an impossible luxury.

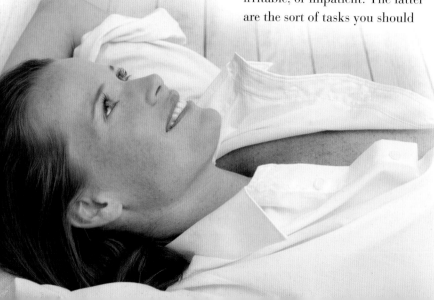

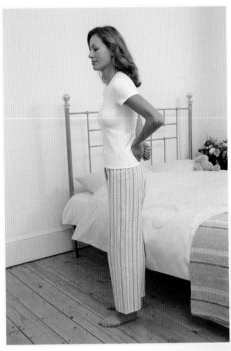

KIDNEY MASSAGE

In Chinese medicine, fear is linked to the energy system of the kidneys, and great importance is placed on keeping this system healthy and flowing naturally. It is therefore a good idea, if you suffer from fear or anxiety in any way, to massage the kidney area vigorously several times during the day, or, at the very least, every morning when you wake up.

1 *Make loose fists, and vigorously (but not too vigorously) tap all around the lower back region – where the kidneys are located.*

2 *Follow this with energetic rubbing. In order to make it have a more far-reaching effect, you may like to send your mind a positive, reinforcing message at the same time:*

"I release fear from my life and am happy to place my trust in the Universe."

Walk not along the paths of fear and mistrust, lest they become your reality

THE KIDNEY AREA

You will find your kidney area by simply placing your hands on either side of your spine, just below your waist – at the top of your buttocks.

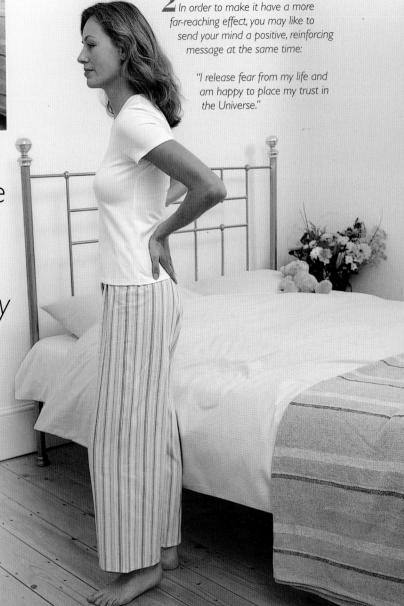

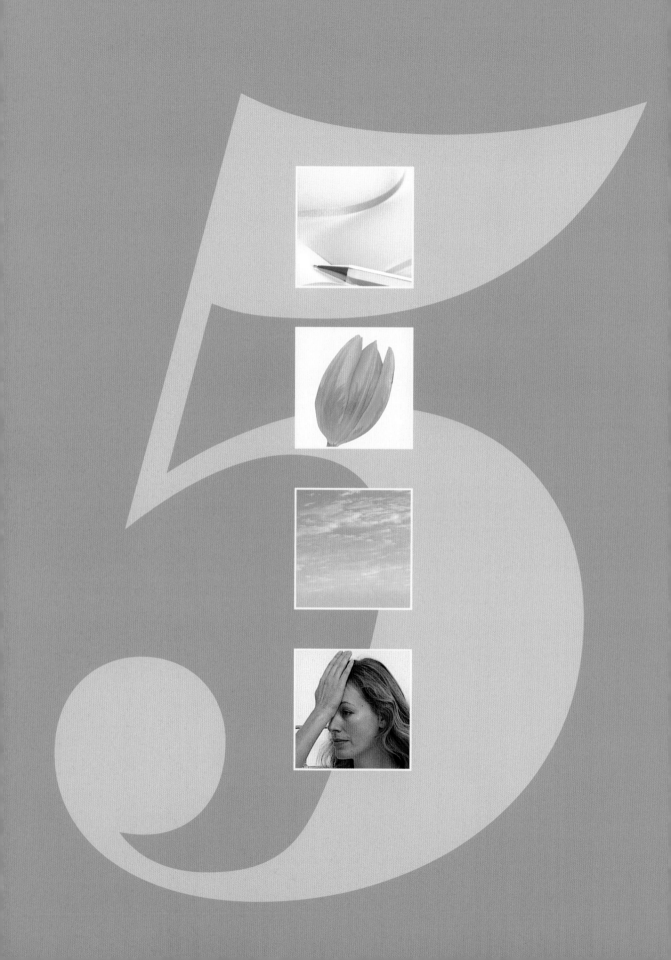

Chapter Five

RELAXING
your way
to sleep

In stilling the mind,

the spirit soars

In stilling the body,

the heart smiles

Clearing your mind

It sometimes seems that the busier we are, the less able we are to switch off. We feel guilty if we're not actually "doing" something, and the body and mind seem to keep going on automatic pilot, looking for complicated answers, when the simplest approaches are often the best.

This is a real indication of an imbalance that can be a main contributor to insomnia, and we need the deeper part of ourselves – the inner sage – to firmly take charge. In the same way that we try to steer our children gently away from destructive habits, we need to do the same for ourselves – especially if these bad habits are leading to a lack of sleep and therefore a continual state of exhaustion.

If you can take a little time to empty your mind before bedtime, you will find that it's much easier to fall asleep. All of the following, very simple, suggestions involve the same underlying principle – finding something positive on which to concentrate, something that will temporarily take you away from disorder and direct you back toward order. When you allow this to happen, you are likely to find that you can have an entirely new perspective: the world around you will miraculously calm down and, in turn, so can you.

To-do lists

It can help to write down the things that you need to do, as one of the most burdensome feelings during a sleepless night is when you have simply forgotten to do something that urgently needs your attention. And for some reason, these things often have a habit of popping into your head in the dead of the night.

★ Write a daily "to do" list for the following day so that all the things to be done tomorrow are, literally, off your mind.

★ Write a weekly "to do" list, so that you know what is likely to need dealing with during the forthcoming week and you can therefore keep on top of things. You will also feel a sense of

USE A NOTEBOOK
Jot down "to do" items in a notebook by your bed.

achievement as you cross them off one by one. It is advisable to prioritize your tasks for the days ahead and to stay realistic about what you can achieve. It is also essential to bring a sense of balance into your week – making spaces in your diary for the things you enjoy, whether meeting friends, planning a family get-together, or going for a walk in the countryside.

★ It can also be a good idea to write a list of the day's (or week's) achievements to remind yourself of all the challenges you have already overcome, rather than getting stuck only on what you haven't yet done. This can help you to feel more at ease, enabling your mind to unwind and sleep to come.

Emotional clear-out

You could also try writing down your problems and difficult feelings to get them off your mind and allow it to shut down during the night. You can destroy the pages if you wish. It's the act of making thoughts into physical reality, by writing them down, that can prove powerful both in settling the mind and in helping you make decisions about what to do next.

"Spontaneous" or "free" writing is worth trying, too. This can prove highly therapeutic as you witness your thoughts taking physical shape on the page in front of you. Try

writing down whatever comes into your mind. It may at first seem incoherent, disordered, and muddled – a disjointed array of random words, or fragments of conversations and events. But as you continue, you will discover that thoughts and feelings begin to flow with a clarity you had not felt before. This can help prevent your thoughts from churning randomly and relentlessly around in your head, which does not make for relaxation or restful sleep.

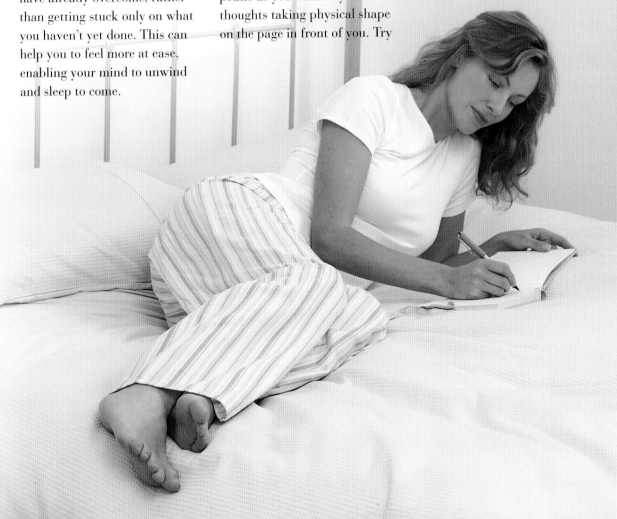

Focus & concentration

There are other effective ways of clearing and steadying the mind in preparation for sleep. Simple focus and concentration is one of them. When tensions are mounting and the world seems to be deteriorating into chaos and ruin, take a few quiet minutes to yourself to try the following exercises.

RELAXING AFTER A HARD DAY

Relax the body as much as you can before doing this exercise, without worrying too much about it – sometimes the harder you try to relax, the more impossible it becomes.

★ *Take your attention to the space between your eyebrows and visualize a blue circle of light there.*

★ *Breathe gently, concentrating on this light until you can allow it to be absorbed inside your head.*

★ *Gently encourage it to move closer to the back of your head, as though it is clearing a space in your mind. Observe its progress.*

★ *Allow it very gently to expand and then disperse throughout your head, clearing your thoughts and your mind, and bringing stillness, calm, and an increased possibility of quality sleep.*

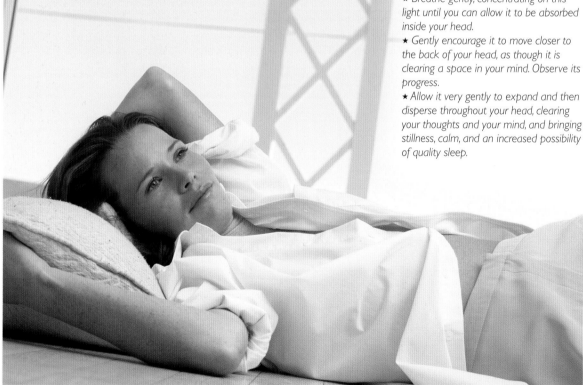

OBJECT-GAZING

Try to come to terms with the fact that you, as a wonderful, created individual, are just as beautiful as the object you are observing during this contemplation.

1 *Find an object of beauty that you enjoy – something from nature, as this will have a balancing effect, helping to still the mind with its natural properties (or energetic vibrations). It could simply be a flower, a leaf, a tree, a gemstone, or perhaps a crystal.*

2 *Gaze at your chosen object, examining it in detail, taking in its colours and the rays of light playing on its surface. Look deeply at it, and then into it, trying to feel the essence of what it is. Try to feel an appreciation of the phenomenal natural forces that brought this object into being. Be aware that these same forces are the ones that brought you into life, and how in this way, we are connected to all things throughout time. Give thanks for these insights and then gently distance yourself from your object. You will probably experience a great feeling of inner peace, so take this with you when you retire for the night.*

Walk the world of wonder from within,
Seek the simple and the gates of heaven
will be open to you,
Walk the way of peace and all will be yours

Breath is Life

Have you ever tried to hold your breath for as long as you possibly can? Or have you ever been swimming under water and thought your lungs would explode from the desperation of needing to breathe? Quality breathing is absolutely crucial to everything we do, including how well we sleep and how much sleep we get.

Breathing is so fundamental to life that we seldom think about it, except when it is threatened in some way, for example by illness or restriction. But without breath, the body would have no fresh supply of its essential fuel – oxygen – and could not survive.

Energy of the heavens

The breath can be used in many ways – whether to stimulate and excite, to facilitate action, to calm and soothe, to focus the mind, to aid concentration, or to relax and heal the body. In the Chinese healing arts it is called the "energy of the heavens" and is valued as a way of transforming external energy (energy from outside us) to internal energy of which we can make use.

The calming breath

Many disciplines, such as yoga and martial arts, use the breath to improve health and stamina, and to direct personal energy, or life force (chi). The breathing techniques and exercises in this chapter not only promote improved health, but also promote deep relaxation, and can therefore be very therapeutic in terms of rest and improved sleep patterns. Good-quality breathing will help to soothe and nourish the nervous system, and correct the imbalances that are so often the cause of sleeplessness in the first place.

All the exercises are designed to bring about a state of calm and relaxation. The key is to gradually work through them, making a mental note of the effects you feel after completing each one, so that you become familiar with how and when each one might be most useful to you. Suggestions are included about when to use each one, but becoming familiar with them yourself is the best way toward understanding the ever-changing needs of your own body.

It is a good idea to heed the Taoist advice on the practice of good breathing habits (see right).

By learning to breathe
you will have life

By learning to breathe well
you will have good health

By learning to breathe deeply
you will live long

By learning to breathe inwardly
you will awaken your immortal spirit

By awakening your immortal spirit
you will breathe into the oneness
of all things

Quality breathing

If you watch a baby or small child, you will notice that their stomach rises and falls with each breath. This is the most natural, tension-free way of breathing, as young children have not learned how to be stressed. It is called "abdominal breathing".

Children only learn more super-ficial, shallow breathing – known as "chest breathing" – later in childhood, largely through copying adults. Ironically, then, we would be better off copying children, as their natural way of breathing is much healthier, as well as more conducive to a relaxed outlook and improved sleep.

Two types of breathing

It is of great benefit to become aware of the difference between the two types of breathing – chest and abdominal – and to retrain yourself to breathe "abdominally". By practising this on a daily basis (see exercise right), you will teach your body to release the stresses and tensions that are all too often the underlying cause of restless or distressed nights.

Chest breathing

We usually find at times of stress, anxiety, and exhaustion that our breathing becomes restricted, being too focused in the upper chest and throat. This shallow "chest breathing" means that we are using less than half our lung capacity with each inward breath. This, in turn, means that insufficient oxygen is entering the blood-stream, resulting in the inefficient clearing and purification of waste products in the blood and major organs. Thus we are, quite literally, starving ourselves of the life force that full and deep breathing can release in us, causing the natural energies to become depleted.

Interestingly, the converse also applies: if we habitually adopt rapid, shallow breathing, then the associated emotions of stress,

tightness, and anxiety are likely to follow (see exercise right). It therefore becomes clear that sustained chest breathing is bound to be detrimental to habitual, good-quality sleep.

Abdominal breathing

The feelings of restriction associated with chest breathing can be brought under control simply by dropping awareness down into the abdomen, until your breathing feels deep and free, and your stomach rises and falls with each inward and outward breath. This correct manner of breathing – known as "abdominal breathing", nourishes your body with a continual supply of fresh oxygen. As your body becomes more relaxed by this, your mind will follow, thus lessening symptoms of stress and making the patterns of disturbed sleep you have fallen into all the easier to resolve.

ABDOMINAL BREATHING

1 *Place your hands on your lower abdomen as a guide and breathe deeply and fully – in a way that makes your abdomen rise and fall with each breath. As you inhale through your nose, allow your abdomen to inflate and your hand to be pushed gently outward.*

2 *As you exhale through the mouth, allow your abdomen to deflate and your hand to sink back in. Continue breathing fully and gently in this way for a few minutes without strain, and then examine how you are feeling in contrast with the chest breathing exercise. You should feel immensely more relaxed.*

CHEST BREATHING

Place your hands on your chest and breathe rapidly into this area. Then think about how it makes you feel. If this is the way you normally breathe you will probably feel the same as usual, but really think deeply about the effects it is having on you. It is probably making you feel stressed, worried, and frantic, without you even knowing it. This type of breathing should generally be avoided.

Breathing Your Way To Sleep

It is especially useful to practise abdominal breathing when you are feeling anxious or tense. It is deeply energizing and relaxing, and you can practise it at any time, whether sitting, standing, moving around, or lying down. Although it may feel a little strange at first, with practice it will soon become easy. Be sure to apply this deep, soothing, abdominal breathing to the range of breathing exercises on the following pages.

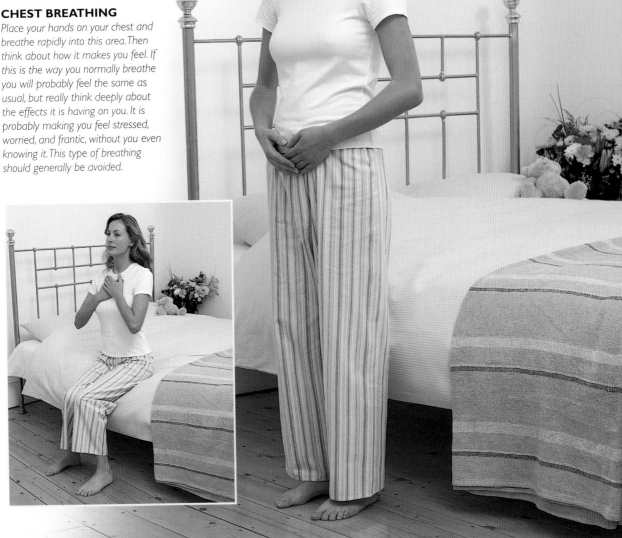

The wise man
sits at rest

An ancient Chinese saying tells us, "Do nothing, and all will be achieved". This breathing exercise lives out this idea, reminding us that all is well when we are in harmony with the natural forces of the universe. It relieves tension and recreates harmony within.

You will feel the benefits of the simple exercise immediately, feeling wonderfully refreshed and relaxed. It can be practised in bed and usually relaxes the body sufficiently for sleep to take place, or at least enough to allow you to switch off a little.

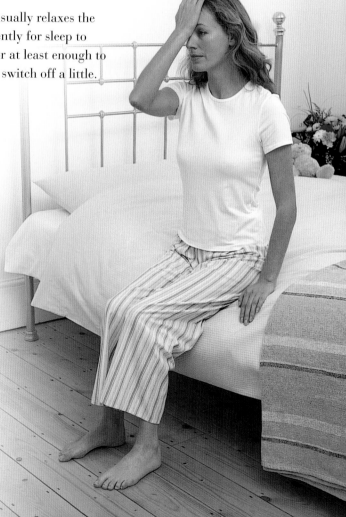

2 *Place the palm of your right hand between your eyebrows. Breathe gently and fully, without strain.*

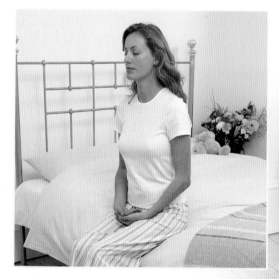

1 *Sit quietly – whether on the floor or a chair – with your back upright. Relax your mind and body and close your eyes. Take a few deep breaths to relax your body even more and increase the level of oxygen in your blood. Place your tongue gently in the roof of your mouth (this may be uncomfortable at first), as this is said to help harmonize the flows of energy within the body, by completing a circuit.*

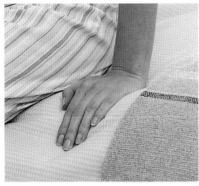

3 *Place the fingertips of your left hand beside you – on the surface upon which you are sitting. Gently press down with the fingers in time with your pulse – listen to your heartbeat to feel its rhythm. Relax into this and continue for a few minutes. You will notice that the speed of your pulse begins to slow down as you breathe in a full and relaxed manner. If unwanted thoughts creep in, simply let them go by, concentrating once more on your heartbeat and breathing.*

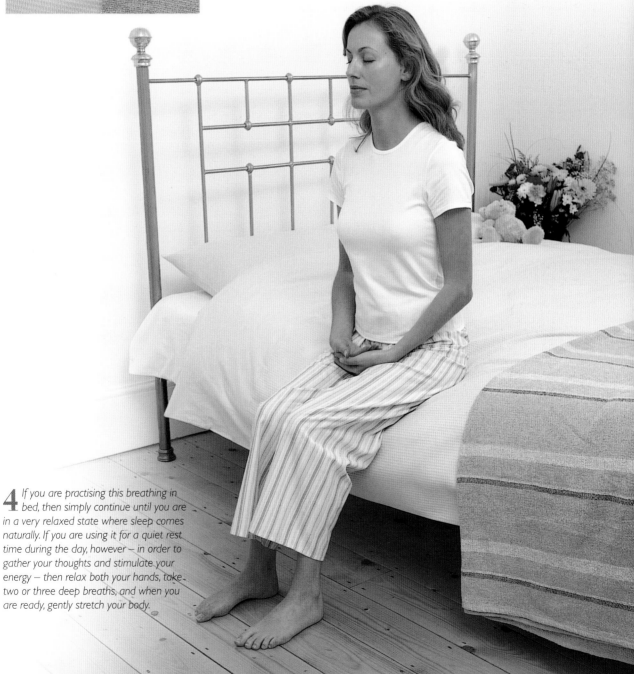

4 *If you are practising this breathing in bed, then simply continue until you are in a very relaxed state where sleep comes naturally. If you are using it for a quiet rest time during the day, however – in order to gather your thoughts and stimulate your energy – then relax both your hands, take two or three deep breaths, and when you are ready, gently stretch your body.*

Completing the circuit

Sometimes, following a period of mental exertion or emotional upheaval, you may feel agitated or unable to clear the mind to think constructively, which can lead to severe disruptions in sleep. This gentle breathing exercise encourages the mind and body to relax through concentration, allowing a natural connection or circuit of energy to take place.

1 *Sit in a relaxed but upright position – whether on the floor, a chair, or your bed.*

This is an excellent exercise to practise at any quiet moment during the day – particularly at times of high tension or anxiety, or late in the evening, before going to bed. It has an extremely beneficial effect on the nervous system, balancing the two sides of the brain (creative and intellectual aspects) and encouraging the mind to become still and clear in order for sleep to come.

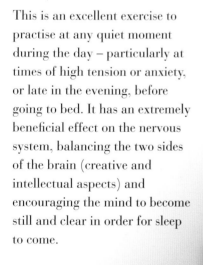

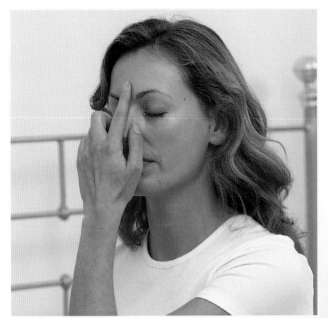

2 Close off one nostril with your thumb and place the index finger of the same hand in the space between your eyebrows. Inhale slowly and deeply through the open nostril, and then exhale through the same nostril. Try to make the in-breath the same length as the out-breath, and allow the breathing to flow naturally, without pauses. Repeat for six breaths.

3 Then use your middle finger to close off the other nostril, simultaneously releasing your thumb from the one closed until now, and keeping your index finger between your eyebrows. Inhale and exhale slowly and gently through the open nostril for six breaths.

Continue steps 2 and 3 for a few minutes. Allow the breath to flow as the waves flow to the shore – not straining or pausing, but moving freely and fully.

Once you have completed your "circuit", simply place your hands in your lap and relax.

The Eagle *awakens*

Stiffness in the body, particularly across the shoulders, can be an indication that tension has been allowed to build, disrupting the body's flow of energy and therefore natural sleeping patterns. Use the image of the eagle's wings to guide the movements in this exercise – strong and sure, yet graceful. Let the movements awaken the body and release tensions.

This is an excellent exercise with which to start and end the day, as it gently works the nervous system, but without a stimulating effect. It is therefore most suitable to be practised before retiring to bed. It is also good for tension headaches arising from muscular aches and pains in the neck and shoulders. As you work through this exercise, visualize the rising and falling of your arms as the wings of an eagle riding the winds – strong and free.

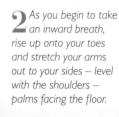

2 As you begin to take an inward breath, rise up onto your toes and stretch your arms out to your sides – level with the shoulders – palms facing the floor.

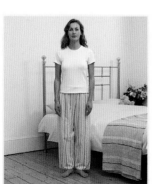

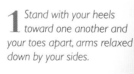

1 Stand with your heels toward one another and your toes apart, arms relaxed down by your sides.

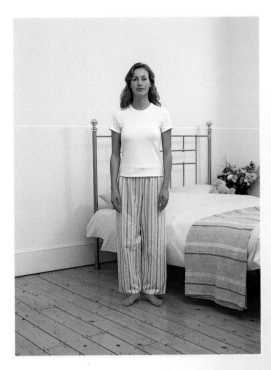

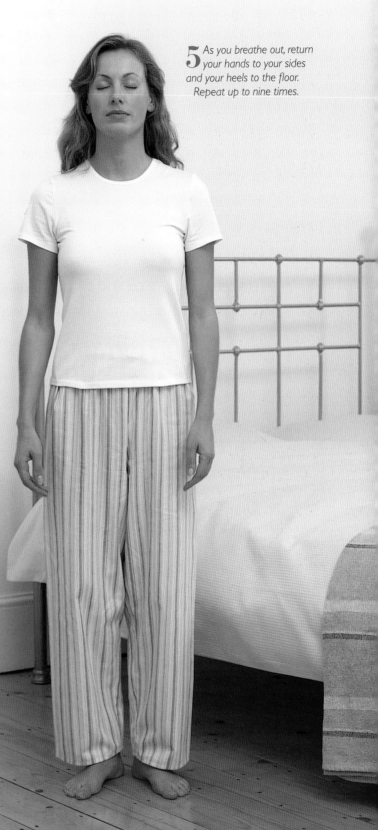

5 *As you breathe out, return your hands to your sides and your heels to the floor. Repeat up to nine times.*

3 Breathing out, lower your arms back to your sides and your heels back onto the floor. Repeat steps 2 and 3 several times, taking full but relaxed breaths.

4 Breathe in as you rise up onto your toes, as before, but this time raise your arms over your head, palms together and stretching upward.

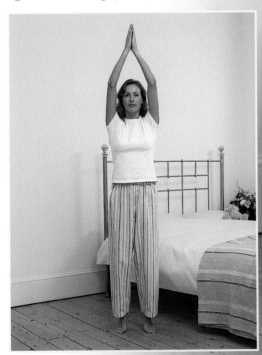

Aligning with heaven & earth

If we align our personal energy flow with the natural energy that flows around us, we will feel as if we are in the right place at the right time. When we are out of harmony, however, life will seem fraught with difficulty. This exercise helps to release excess and stagnant energy, thus generally rebalancing us.

This gentle stretching exercise is of particular benefit after sitting or standing for a long period of time, as it refreshes the whole body and redistributes energy, encouraging it to start flowing harmoniously once again. Try it at the end of a taxing day: as it refreshes the body, so it enables the body to relax and shrug off stress and tension. As you do it, imagine you are able to draw heaven down through the crown of your head, and the earth up through the soles of your feet.

2 Bring your palms together in front of you – in a low prayer position.

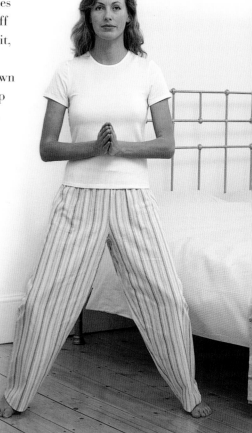

1 Stand with your feet wide apart and parallel, your knees a little bent, and your hands rested on your thighs. In order to straighten your back, slightly draw your stomach up, and release your tailbone downward. Take a breath, keeping it low in your abdomen.

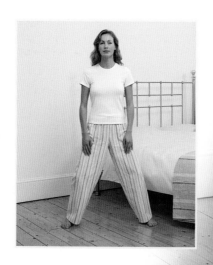

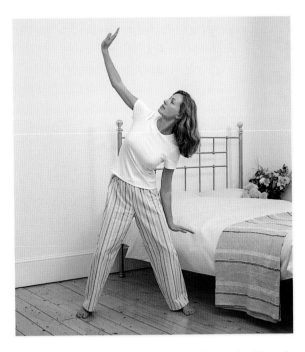

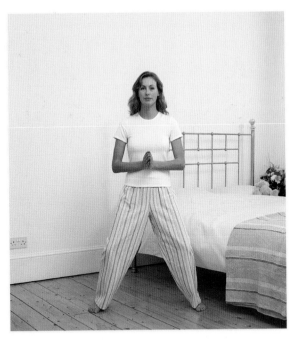

3 As you breathe out, raise your right hand up to the right, palm toward the ceiling, and at the same time, lower your left hand down to the left, palm toward the floor. Feel a stretch along your arms, and lift your head to look at your raised hand.

4 Breathe in to bring your palms back down to where you started – in front of you and together.

5 As you breathe out again, raise and lower the opposite hand from step 3, again looking at your raised hand and stretching along your arms.
Breathe in to bring your palms together in front of you.

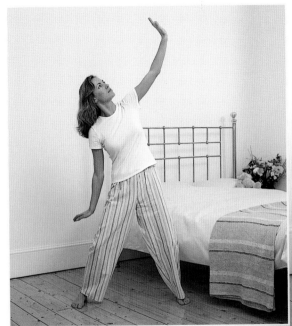

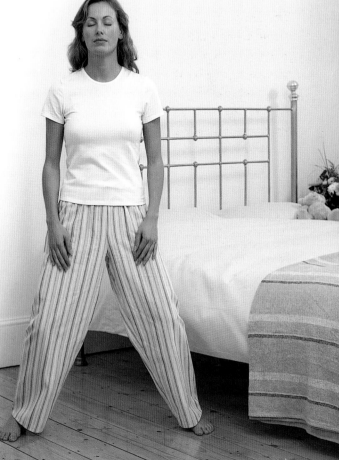

Calming the *dragon*

It is said that when there is an excess of fire in the energy system, heat rises through the body, making sleep seem almost impossible. This exercise helps to calm this Yang energy, releasing the Dragon's Breath, and encouraging recuperative Yin energy.

The sound "haaaa" is the Chinese healing sound for the heart and the heart energy system. This deeply relaxing exercise causes a vibration, which sets up a positive and balancing healing throughout this system. It is thought that excess energy here is one of the primary causes of insomnia. It is therefore a very suitable exercise to perform before going to bed, and indeed at any time during the day when stress threatens to take over, or tempers and nerves become frayed. Each time you breathe out "haaaa", imagine you are releasing the powerful breath of the dragon.

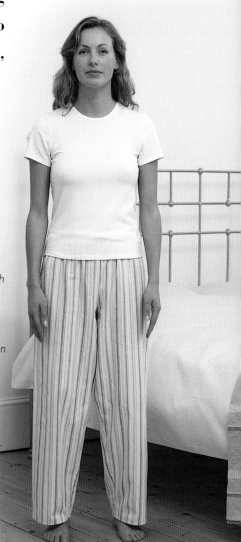

1 *Stand with your feet shoulder-width apart, hands down by your sides, and the body relaxed, but upright. Breathe deeply into your abdomen, letting go of each breath with a "haaaa" sound. Allow anger and tension to be dissolved by this exhaling sound.*

Look within to seek the Dragon Breathe with a calmness of spirit And his fiery breath will be quenched

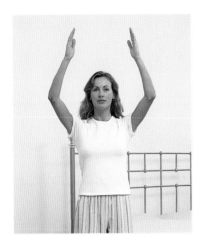

2 Breathe in, and raise your hands above your head.

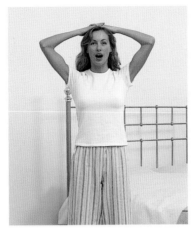

3 Breathe out as you link your fingers and lower your hands onto the crown of your head, making the sound "haaaa" with the exhalation. Then breathe in.

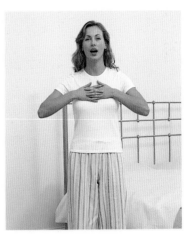

4 Breathing out with the "haaaa" sound, slowly lower your hands onto your chest. Then breathe in.

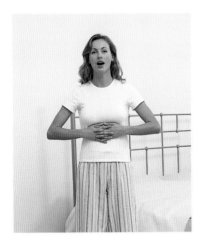

5 Breathe out ("haaaa"), and lower your hands, with the fingers still linked, to the space between your lower ribs. Breathe in.

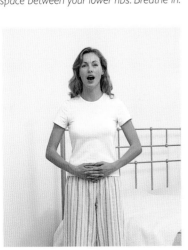

6 Breathe out ("haaaa"), and lower your hands down on to your abdomen area – the Tan Tien (see p. 29). Breathe in.

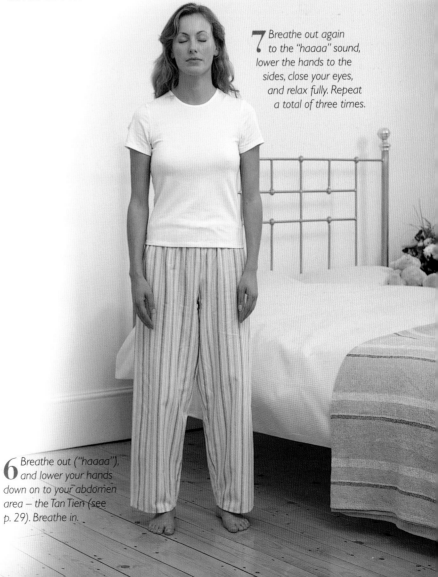

7 Breathe out again to the "haaaa" sound, lower the hands to the sides, close your eyes, and relax fully. Repeat a total of three times.

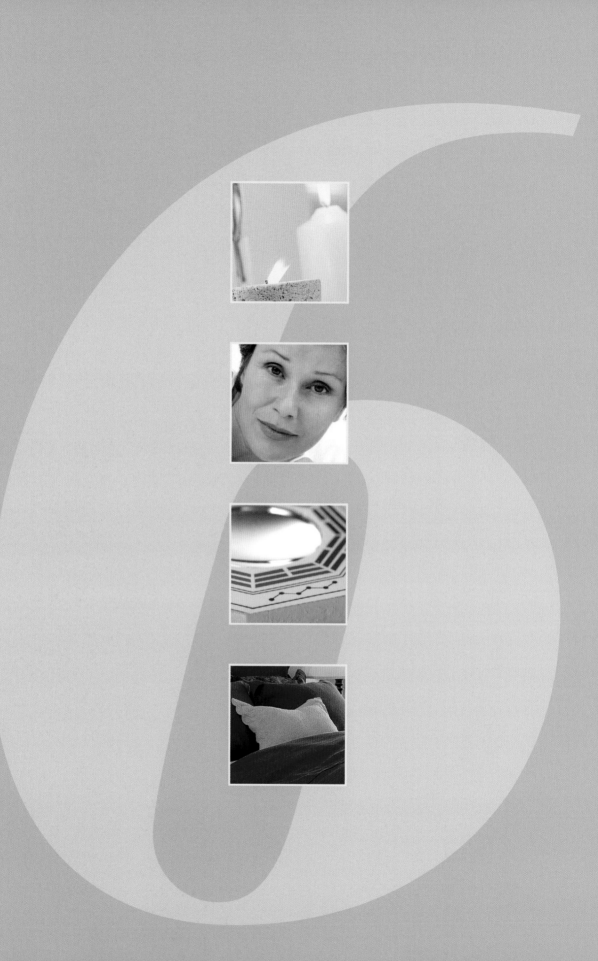

Chapter Six

Healing your
SLEEPING SPACE

The gods dwell within sacred walls and watch over us while we sleep

The art of feng shui

Chi is the "universal energy" that breathes life into us and our surroundings. Healers first acknowledged the importance of being in harmony with this flow thousands of years ago, and Ancient Chinese philosophers concluded that by making changes in our surroundings, we could change the energy flow around us, and thus our health and fortune. A complex healing art thus evolved, known as Feng Shui, which entails harmonizing each person's surroundings to suit them.

Feng shui helps many people the world over make decisions regarding the interior of their home. The principles can be applied to the whole home or to individual rooms. In this book, we will explore ideas for healing your sleeping space, thereby improving the quality of your sleep and rest time.

In balance?

Feng shui – literally meaning wind and water – is a Chinese philosophy that takes account of nature's elements – metal, water, wood, fire, and earth – and states that everyone has a dominant element in their personal make-up, according to the season of their birth. But the terms wind and water could also be considered symbolically: wind representing the wind of change – inevitable in life, whether a gentle breeze or a mighty tempest; and water symbolizing the other fundamental element of life – nourishing energy and movement toward growth. These two aspects, when harnessed in a positive way, produce far-reaching results.

If our surroundings are in harmony with these natural, life-giving forces, then it follows that we, too, will be able to directly benefit, and enjoy good health and blessings. However, if we are in some way at odds with our surroundings, and our life force is adversely affected, our health and well-being will also suffer.

"The Way"

Fundamental to this philosophy is the belief that all life comes from the same infinite source. In this sense, we are connected to the whole of creation. Life flows from, and returns to, the source. This is "The Way", or the Tao, and from this comes the term, Taoism – the ancient Chinese philosophy upon which most of the information in this book is based. In order for our lives to flourish with health and fortune, it must be in harmony with the infinite forces of nature – for this is "The Way".

Yin and yang

From this perspective, life is a balance – a balance between two opposing forces, Yin and Yang. Yin is the feminine principle of life and describes the inward-looking aspects of ourselves, which are seeking answers. Yang, on the other hand, is the masculine principle, which takes creative and resourceful action. Yin is equated with manifestations of energy such as night, darkness, cold, introspection, intuition, earth, the moon, softness, and stillness. Yang is equated with manifestations of energy

such as, light, daytime, sun, male, creative, heat, action, and heaven. Insomnia is often an indication that Yang energy has become too dominant and there is little room for the Yin of rest, recovery, gentleness, and intuition.

By learning to harness the forces of Yin, which is viewed as earth energy, we will find that we are more readily able to achieve quality rest, thus becoming more effective at our daytime tasks and more insightful in our thoughts.

Author's Advice

It can be useful to think of the process of inner exploration, growth and development as being a form of personal feng shui in that inner growth can be made possible by looking at a particular emotional problem or challenge, and simply making the practical alterations necessary to resolve it. This will alter the flow of chi and allow positive change to take place, thus encouraging a positive change in our sleeping patterns. After all, it becomes impossible to continue in the same way if both your body and mind are exhausted.

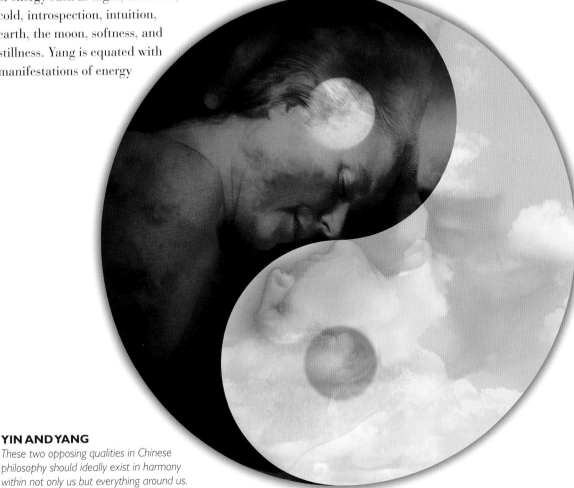

YIN AND YANG
These two opposing qualities in Chinese philosophy should ideally exist in harmony within not only us but everything around us.

Feng shui for restful sleep

Insomnia can be an indication that the natural needs for rest and recuperation are not being met and supported by our surroundings. It might therefore be the case that an area of disharmony in the home, or, in particular the bedroom or sleeping area, needs realigning in order to emanate the maximum amount of positive energy and to bring it into a Yin–Yang balance.

SETTING THE SCENE
Lighting several candles in your bedroom not only makes for a romantic setting, but also creates a generally relaxing atmosphere.

The aim of feng shui is not only to facilitate this, but also to change the nature of harmful energy – sometimes known as sha chi – so that it no longer has an adverse effect. The premise is that if our surrounding energies are in harmony with the infinite, our personal energies will also be encouraged to respond in this way. There are numerous feng shui "remedies" to achieve this.

Sometimes, simple adjustments can bring about huge changes, and this is something we should all be confident enough to address in our own homes.

Home sweet home

Your home should primarily be a haven – somewhere you feel safe, secure, and as private as you wish. It should be somewhere you enjoy spending time and you look forward to coming back to. Whether large or small, permanent or temporary, your home should ideally be an expression of yourself. In the same way that the style in which you choose to dress or the kind of occupation you choose to undertake should be a creative expansion of your innermost self, so too should your home. If you feel in any way uncomfortable there, then you need to make some changes.

The boudoir

Let us turn our attention to the bedroom – the room most relevant to insomnia. The first thing to ascertain in order to harmonize this area is whether or not you actually like the room and feel comfortable being there. Go through the self-questioning process on pages 92–93 to gain valuable insight into how your current sleeping environment is affecting your state of being. Remember that there are no such things as "wrong" answers to these questions. The worst that can happen is that the energy will stay the same as before, and the best is that your sleeping patterns – and therefore life – will be completely transformed – for the good.

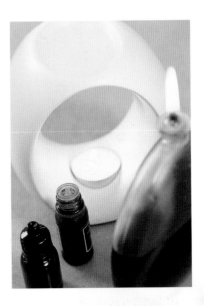

SOOTHING SCENTS

You can improve the energetic feel of a room by infusing it with a soothing scent of your choice. A good way to do this is to burn an essential oil (see pp. 100–107) in a specially designed oil burner.

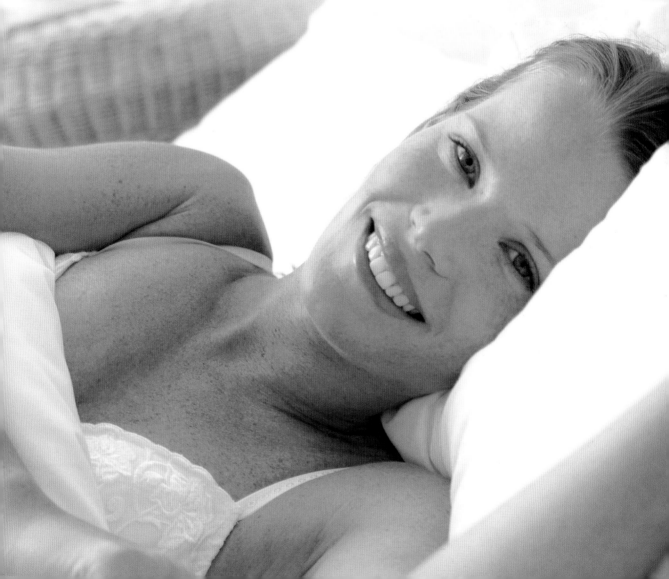

Do I like this room**?**

Your bedroom should provide you with a comfortable, peaceful area, which supports your changing needs. By following the simple guidelines that follow, a harmonious atmosphere can be created, encouraging a flow of relaxing energy, where rest and sleep can take place. This is your sacred space, where you can truly be yourself.

★ Stand a little distance from the open door and take a good look into the room. What do you think of what you see?

★ Take a step forward to the threshold and observe how that feels to you.

★ Now step into the room and

Shared Space

It is important to create an ambience that is pleasing and relaxing to all occupants of the bedroom. If your needs and tastes are very much at odds with those of your partner or room mate, and it is adversely affecting one of you, then you should discuss the possibilities: you might either find décor that pleases and soothes both of you or you might decide that having separate sleeping spaces would be better.

observe your feelings and your energy. Does the room feel warm and welcoming, cold and unwelcoming, or fairly neutral? Does your energy expand or drop when you walk through the door? And if you close your eyes, are these feelings accentuated?

★ Walk over to your bed and observe how you are feeling and how your energy is reacting. Ask yourself whether or not you feel happy and comfortable.

★ Lie down on the bed and again observe any changes in your energy. Do not rush this – be prepared to spend a little time, perhaps repeating the process over a few days and making notes of your findings.

★ Have a thorough and honest look around the room. Often the most obvious feature to observe is the colour. Is it one that you

particularly like, dislike, or is it someone else's choice, and you just feel that it will "do"?

★ Do you like the furniture and the way your clothing is stored? Are you making best use of your space? Are your curtains and bedding to your liking? If you have ornaments or knick-knacks, do you like them, or have they just been there for years, so that you hardly see them anymore? Do you have pictures or posters on the walls that make you feel good?

Yes, I like it

Ideally, you should like your room very much and feel totally at ease there – somewhere to relax, unwind, and rest after the day's events. It should provide you with a sanctuary where you can reflect and contemplate,

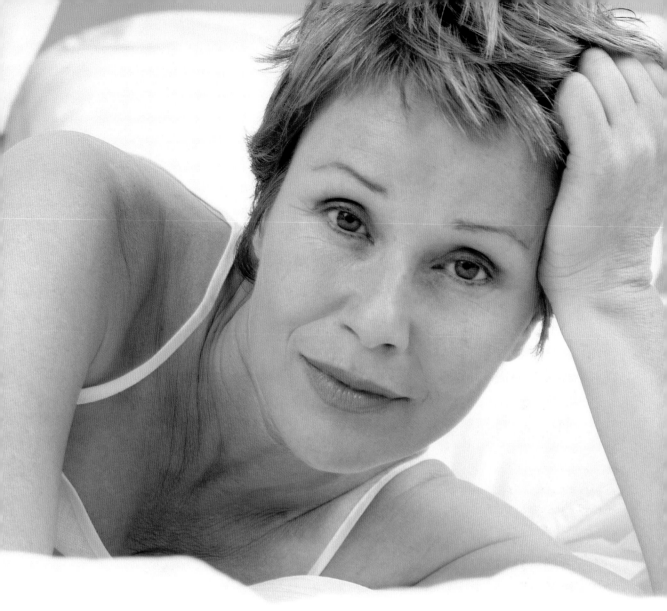

and it should emanate a gentle, restful energy. The impression should be of flowing peace and tranquillity, and the colours, shapes, furniture, and accessories, should echo this. If all of this is the case, it is unlikely to be any aspect of your room that is causing your insomnia.

No, I hate it

If you feel in any way uncomfortable, drained, depleted, agitated, anxious, depressed, or sad in your sleeping surroundings, then action needs to be taken. This is an opportunity to make changes to anything in the room that you dislike, because by disliking something, you send negative energy toward it, blocking the flow of positive energy desired. See pages 94–99 for a range of factors to consider changing.

However, if you still cannot reconcile yourself to your room after making all the suggested changes, you may have to consider changing the use of the rooms in your home, so that you can sleep in a room that feels better suited to your needs.

Tune Into Your Own Needs

Remember that the best guide, in terms of creating a harmonious and restful sleeping space, is you. You know your own likes and dislikes, what you find relaxing, and what disturbs you. The art of energy healing, whether on an emotional level, or in terms of living space, is very much to do with listening to your needs, acknowledging what brings you pleasure or pain, and making changes and adjustments, with these as your guide.

The principles *of* *feng shui*

The following feng shui principles are the main factors that can influence the energy – or lack thereof – in your sleeping space, so think about each one in connection to your own room and then make the changes most likely to help you sleep.

Colour

The colour of your bedroom can play a large part in whether or not the room has a restful atmosphere. Bright, vibrant colours can prove to be rather too stimulating, whereas softer shades – blues, greens, violets, pinks, creams – create more of a feeling of peace. Pastel colours are the ideal colour to aid sleep, as they take the body into a peaceful, introspective state, and help to slow a racing mind. Some people find it helpful to use a low-wattage blue bulb to relax the body and allow sleep to come. Blue is the colour of peace and dreams. However, if the room is north-facing, blue may look a little too cold and a warmer colour may be necessary, such as a soft green, pink, or cream. Green can be particularly good as it introduces a feeling of nature and harmonious balance, while pink or apricot would bring about a feeling of love and well-being. Blue could still be introduced in the form of something like a blue bulb in a side light.

Furniture

It is crucial to have furniture around you that you both like and find useful. Do not put up with something just because you feel obliged to keep it, as it will attract stagnating energy. Every time you look at it you will send it some sort of bad "vibe" or negative thought, cutting it off from the flow of positive energy that you are aiming to develop in the room. So, remove everything you do not actively like or use: sell it, give it away, or throw it away. Your room will instantly feel transformed and lighter.

Accessories

If your sleeping space is to be your ideal haven, it should include accessories that reflect your tastes and preferences, and which can help to enhance feelings of comfort and security in order to promote sleep.

Try to limit straight lines and angles in your bedroom by softening harsh corners – perhaps with the use of drapes and cushions. Introduce curved shapes, and textures that bring

COLOUR SCHEMES

Choose your bedroom shades from the pastel end of the spectrum. Softer hues create an atmosphere of peace and pastel colours are conducive to sleep.

about feelings of comfort – huge pillows, a rug to sink your toes into, plush, rounded cushions, and a large duvet or bedcover to mould around the contours of your body. Put up pictures or photographs of people you love. Go for comfort in a big way.

Bed placement

The placement of the bed is seen to be of paramount importance in feng shui. Ideally, the bed should not be directly against a wall if there are two people sleeping in it, as both people should be free to climb in and out on different sides. The bed should not block the opening of wardrobe doors or drawers, and should not either be directly under a window or be directly facing a window, as the flow of energy will be too rapid. At one time, it was believed to be bad luck to place the bottom of the bed facing the door, as this is the position in which the dead are

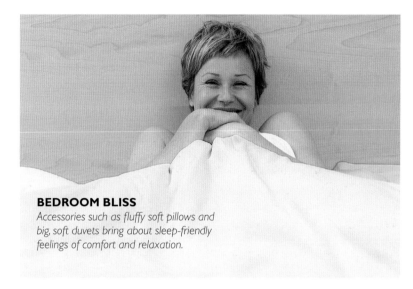

BEDROOM BLISS
Accessories such as fluffy soft pillows and big, soft duvets bring about sleep-friendly feelings of comfort and relaxation.

laid. These days, however, it is considered more important to move your bed away from the door simply to avoid draughts.

It is also considered, in the practice of feng shui, to be inauspicious to lie under a ceiling beam. It is thought that your body's energy may become segmented while you sleep, leading to headaches and difficulty waking in the morning. If possible, move the bed to a

position between any beam-like structures. However, if you are unable to do this, either place your feet (rather than your head) under a beam, or try softening them with hanging drapes.

Positioning the bed east–west seems to have a relaxing effect, enhancing the quality of sleep. The best placement for the bed, then, is diagonally opposite the door, in an east–west direction, giving a good view of the whole room, and leaving space around it for air circulation.

Try to arrange the existing furniture with your bed as a centrepiece and the other furniture placed all around it, and angled across corners, if possible. This is because chi naturally flows in curves and gets lost or stagnant in empty corners. Attempting to soften corners, using as much of them as possible, and cleaning them regularly is therefore extremely good practice.

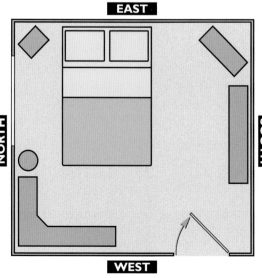

DESIGNING YOUR BEDROOM
In Feng Shui terms, the position of your bed is of paramount importance. Positioning it east–west has a relaxing effect and placing it neither directly under nor facing a window avoids a restless, rapid flow of energy around the room.

The power of sound

Sound is another carrier of energy, as it produces specific vibrations. You may like to introduce pleasing sounds to your sleeping space, bearing in mind that they should not intrude upon your rest. A gentle wind chime hanging in the garden can produce a wonderfully comforting sound at night, as can a water feature, but you must be guided by your own preferences – some people like perfect silence at night-time, while others prefer to be soothed by natural sounds.

Heaven scent

Flat, or negative, feelings in your room can be dispersed with the aid of essential oils. A spray mist can be made using a few drops of natural aromatic oils (see pp. 104–107) and water, or scented candles can be used to create a warm and welcoming atmosphere. However, make sure that any candles you use are made from beeswax and that they are only scented with essential oils, which are natural fragrances. This will ensure that they do not give off any toxic vapours, which may further disturb the energy of the room.

External factors

Certain external factors – over which you feel you have no power – may have a bearing on your room. There may be a telegraph pole looming at your window, or a large, gloomy tree or building cutting off most of your natural light, or a view that you simply do not like. In these instances, an effective remedy is to hang a small crystal or mirror outside the window. This serves to redirect the disturbing energy away from your room. If it is something like street lights or the noise of traffic that is disturbing you, try to invent some pleasing means of blocking out the light or noise. Otherwise, the last course of action should be moving to another room, as the importance of good-quality sleep should not be underestimated.

SOOTHING SOUNDS
Hanging a windchime either in or somewhere near the bedroom can provide just the thing some people need to help lull them off to sleep.

Crystal clear

Keep ornaments and accessories to a minimum in the bedroom,

particularly crystals, which have become very popular in recent years. Crystals are powerful projectors and magnifiers of energy which, despite being great in other areas of the home, can often prove too disturbing in a bedroom. If you want to have crystals around you, it's best to seek professional advice as to which ones have a good reso-nance with your personal energy at the time and remember that this will keep changing, so be prepared to be flexible. A rose quartz would be the best general bet for the bedroom, though, as the colour pink helps to generate soothing heart energy. It, like all crystals, would have to be regularly charged and cleansed, as they tend to absorb and magnify energy in their immediate environment. The best way to do this is to place them in direct sunlight for several hours every so often.

Is the room free from clutter?

Have a good look around – what is in the corners, under the bed,

ROSE QUARTZ
Pink is the colour of peaceful, loving, heart energy. This makes a rose quartz the ideal choice if you would like to place a crystal somewhere in your bedroom to help create a calm ambience, conducive to sound sleep.

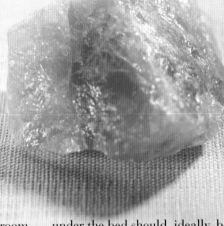

behind the door? Does the room feel spacious, light, and airy, or is it cluttered with so much stuff that it's hard to think straight as soon as you enter it?

Clutter attracts negative chi. This is because it disrupts harmonious flow, particularly if it is clutter that is seldom touched or dealt with. Energy is allowed to stagnate around the clutter because it is unable to flow freely. The bedroom should therefore be as clear as possible. Avoid having piles of laundry, paperwork, and empty cups everywhere. Instead, special places should be found for clothes and dirty laundry should be kept out of sight. The space

under the bed should, ideally, be kept clear, again to allow energy – and air – to circulate freely. The room should be cleaned regularly and kept fresh.

Is there electrical equipment?

Electronic equipment should not be kept in the bedroom. And if it is, any screens should be kept covered and plugs should be unplugged when the devices are not in use. This even applies to items as small as hairdryers.

This is because they emit positive ions that can have a detrimental effect on our health – an electrical charge that can make us feel irritable and nervous. If it is unavoidable to keep these in the sleeping area, they should be as far away from the bed as possible and turned away at an angle. Placing a quartz crystal in the area of the screen will help to nullify the

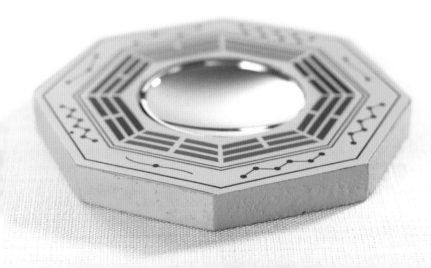

WARD AWAY EVIL SPIRITS
Feng shui talismans are freely available these days. These small, often patterned, carved, or engraved objects are thought to have protective powers.

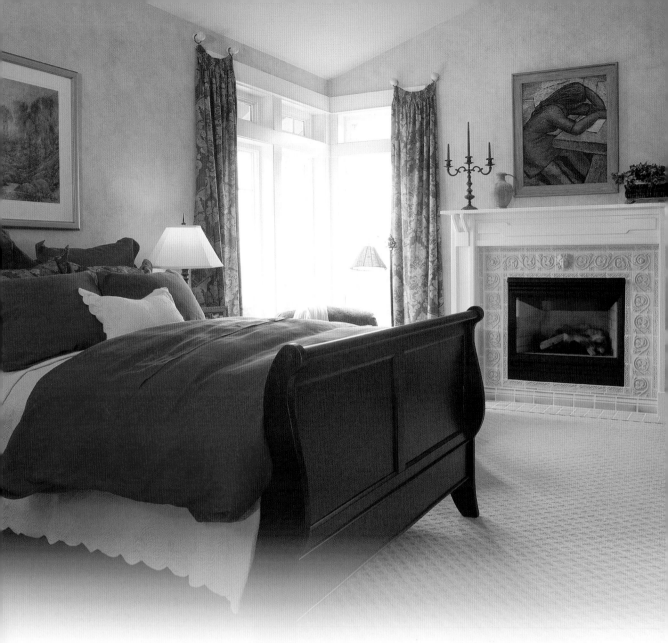

negative effects, as will the use of an ionizer (these devices are usually available from your local hardware store). This is particularly relevant if you also work in an environment where a lot of electrical equipment is used. In this case, you are probably even more in need of a break from these conditions, which makes it all the more important to relocate the electrical goods.

If lack of space is a problem, then screening-off an area in your bedroom for items like computers and televisions is a good alternative. You could use something as simple as a light drape or curtain to do this. This will reinforce the idea that rest and relaxation are in no way dependent on external stimuli, but must come from within. It is never a good idea, for example, to habitually use the television to lull you off to sleep. This is not true relaxation, as it leaves you with a buzz of too much stimulation, rather than the peace and tranquillity desired.

Is there sufficient ventilation and daylight?

Fresh air and natural daylight are the very best ways of creating positive energy in your environment, as they are natural sources of positive energy.

During the daytime, always allow as much light into your room as you can – throwing your curtains back and opening the blinds. Leaving a window open for a little while every day will recharge the room with positive chi, in preparation for the next night. It is also a good idea to leave a window open while you sleep, if possible, as this will let fresh air circulate and prevent stuffiness from building up, especially if more than one person is sleeping in the room.

When there is little natural daylight available, such as in a basement, use other remedies, such as aroma, sound, colour, and furniture placement, to create a supportive environment for yourself, stimulating the energy into positive flow.

If the energy in the room feels rather flat, then hanging a faceted crystal in the window will enliven it during the daytime. Any sunlight will catch it and send rainbows dancing around the room, creating powerfully positive chi.

Where are the mirrors in the room?

The use and placement of mirrors in a room can completely alter the energy of the space. The energy of images bouncing off a mirror will be magnified. It is, therefore, of great importance to place any mirrors in a way that they will not magnify or project an image that you do not want to introduce – such as a dreary view or a cluttered corner. Equally, you do not want to magnify energy in a way that produces a rush of overly fast-flowing chi. For example, magnifying a window, or another mirror, may be fine in a living space, but often proves

too enlivening for an area of sleep and recuperation. It is also inadvisable to reflect the entrance to the room, as this projects energy out of the room, leaving the room depleted and cut off.

According to ancient wisdom, it is also highly inadvisable – to the point of folly – to place a mirror in an area that reflects people sleeping. This is because it is thought that, during the night, the energy bodies separate from the physical body – particularly during dreams –

and that the reflection of the sleeping body may provide confusion as you strive to realign on waking – leaving you feeling sleepy, disturbed, or disjointed. Mirrors placed in this way can also provoke disturbed dreams for the same reason.

Unless you have a large bedroom and can place a mirror in a neutral place which will not activate or deflect too much energy, then the ideal position for a mirror is on the inside of a cupboard door.

Feng Shui Summary

Below is a quick reminder of the main feng shui principles that insomnia sufferers should apply to their bedroom or sleeping space in order to make it as rest- and sleep-friendly as possible.

★ *Choose a colour that you like, and which is conducive to rest.*
★ *Place the furniture in as close to a circular positioning as you can in the room, as chi does not follow straight lines, but curves and spirals. Corners should be softened to help this flow – in particular by placing items of furniture diagonally across them.*
★ *The bed should be placed in view of, but not in direct line with, either the door or the windows, and should face east–west if possible. You may need to try different alignments until you find the one that most suits you.*
★ *Place mirrors inside cupboards.*
★ *Remove anything – furniture or otherwise – that you do not really like or that serves no purpose. It is important to be soothed and pleased by your surroundings.*
★ *Be ruthless about removing rubbish and clutter from your bedroom,*
including that which occupies drawers and cupboards – it does not have to be visible to have a detrimental effect. You will be surprised by how much better you feel once you have pared everything down to a minimum. It will feel as though a weight has been lifted. Then make sure you keep the area well cleaned and tidy.
★ *Relocate computers and televisions to other rooms in your house. If this is not possible, then cover with screens when not in use – particularly at night. Use an ionizer, a quartz crystal, and natural daylight to combat the harmful effects of electronic equipment.*
★ *Make sure that your room is well ventilated at all times and that as much light as possible floods the room during the day. This will help to re-energize it for the coming night.*

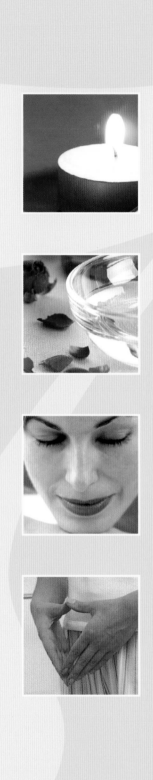

Chapter Seven

Using
ESSENTIAL
OILS

Inhale the healing aromas,

Soak up the soothing scents,

Bathe in the beauty,

And be at peace

The beauty of aromatherapy

The art of using aromatic extracts from plants and tree resins to bring about balance and healing is an ancient one, which has enjoyed a strong revival in recent years. When we buy brightly packaged oils from store shelves, we are making use of the knowledge of ages past – an art that has evolved over time into what is known today as "aromatherapy".

Even the more unusual essential oils are becoming readily available these days, although some should not be used without specialist knowledge (see below).

Choose Carefully

Some plant extracts can lead to toxic build up if used excessively, so should be used sparingly and with care. Advice should be sought from a qualified aromatherapist if you are in any doubt about the safety of the oil that you are considering using. However, as a general guideline, the ones that are readily available can be used quite safely, as long as the instructions are followed. Synthetic oils, such as perfume oils – distinct from essential oils – should not be used for healing because they have no therapeutic value, and are really just superficial perfumes.

Always look for pure plant extracts and be sure that they are suitable for the purpose you have in mind, whether for relaxation or stimulation of the senses. Different therapeutic plants have very differing attributes (or energetic vibrations), which influence their nature and the effect they have on the human energy field. In fact, specialist photography techniques allow us to see the changes in the aura of an individual when an essential oil is introduced, either onto the skin, or into the energy field via a spray or burner.

How oils work

Essential oils can be used purely for the pleasure of the beautiful aromas they give off, or for more medicinal purposes: to help bring about balance on all levels – mind, body, and spirit. Although we are tempted to consider ourselves purely as dense, physical bodies, the vibrations of essential oils actually work through our more subtle aspects – our chi, or life force, before moving into the physical body, to bring about physiological changes. For example, a tree resin might offer strengthening and enduring vibrations via its fragrance, while those of a rose will be more relaxing and immediately beautiful. And certain oils are particularly beneficial in the treatment of insomnia as they have inherent soothing or soporific vibrations (see pp. 104–107).

As with all vibrational remedies, the more open the recipient, the stronger the effects will be. This is because, the mind has the power to direct the flow of energy, or chi, and can therefore also either block out or enhance the energy of any subtle or vibrational therapy.

The power of scent

Smells often evoke emotional responses in us: we find ourselves being very drawn to some things – whether the smell of newly mown grass, freshly baked bread, a field of lavender, or a garden of roses. Equally, there are smells that some people really dislike, such as tar, petrol, or fish, and which provoke an emotional response of revulsion or disgust. Our sense of smell could thus be thought of as a pathway to our feelings, which, in turn, provides a pathway to the spiritual side of our being. For this reason, essential oils can have an immensely therapeutic effect on those who choose to use them. After all, our sense of smell is one of our most treasured senses – indeed, the first one to develop in a growing baby. The many varied scents of the oils can therefore have all sorts of effects, including soporific ones if the right oils are chosen, which can help restore healthy sleeping patterns.

How To Use Oils

There are many effective ways to introduce essential oils into your daily life to make the most of their therapeutic effect.. Below is a list of the main methods that are useful when trying to remedy the exhaustion and lethargy created by insomnia.

★ ***Burn it:*** *Add half a dozen drops of your chosen essential oil (see pp. 104–107) to water, and burn in an oil burner to fragrance the room.*

★ ***Spray it:*** *A fragranced room-spray can be made by adding a few drops of essential oils to water. This can be very useful for raising the quality of vibrations in a room and also for just misting lightly into your energy field, around your head and body.*

★ ***Soak in it:*** *A warm and relaxing evening bath is extremely enjoyable. Simply add about five or six drops of oil and relax for about twenty minutes,* *inhaling the wonderful aromas, and allowing the mind to let go of the tensions of the day. This is particularly soothing just before you go to bed and should help you relax into a deep sleep.*

★ ***Lie on it:*** *Sprinkle a few drops of oil on your bed sheets or pillows so that you breathe it in as you try to drift off.*

★ ***Rub it in:*** *Using essential oils to give a massage is greatly soothing and is likely to relax you deeply and help you nod off to sleep (see pp. 108–111).*

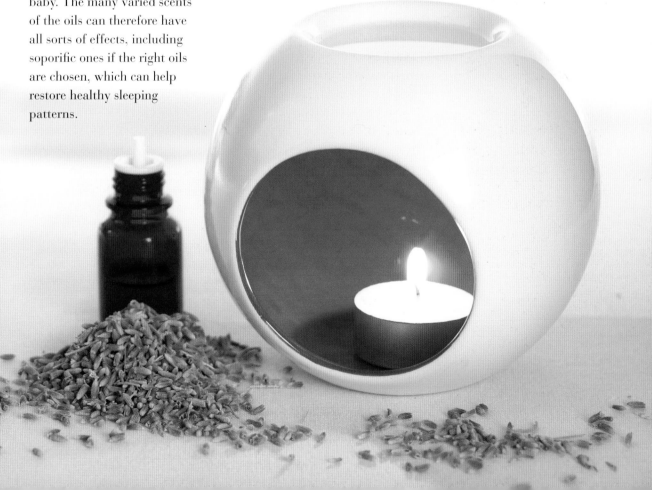

Essential oils *for* insomnia

A beautiful aroma is one of the most wonderful ways in which to nourish the spirit and calm the mind in order to lull you into a deep and refreshing sleep. Allow yourself the time to bask in the luxury of the oils of your choice – your mind relaxing and letting go of the worries of the day, and your body resting, recuperating, and restoring itself to balance.

There are, of course, numerous essential oils that may be helpful in promoting relaxation and sleep. The following are just some of the most readily available which will help to release the emotional aspects playing a part in your inability to sleep. Most health stores should stock a wide range of oils, but always check that the ones you are buying are pure plant extracts – organic where possible.

Benzoin
This oil is made from the scented resin of a large tropical tree – *Styraz benzoin*. It is warming, strengthening, and relaxing, thus encouraging us to let go of the fretting of an overactive mind and potentially promoting more restful sleep. Its strengthening qualities can also provide the space for us to acknowledge and release past emotional traumas and feelings of being burdened or overloaded.

The colour released by this oil into the aura is a rich and warming red, having the effect of awakening our connection to the earth and the physical world. This aspect is often under-developed in modern society, where much of our living is by artificial means and based around the workings of the mind. Allow the red of this oil to penetrate the energy field and help you to relax into being reconnected to life.

Bergamot
The properties of this oil – which is extracted from the bergamot tree (*Citrus bergamia*) – have a special affinity with the heart. Its light fragrance can bring joy, comfort, and laughter into even the most difficult circumstances. It gives us the confidence to ask for help and guidance, and the courage to look past the dark-ness into our own unique light. It also awakens the heart, allowing us to reach out with a lightness of spirit to people, and helps us view challenges with a new perspective, seeing the light, rather than the shadows.

This oil is connected with two colours: the light sunshine yellow, which signifies connecting to life with optimism, and dispelling gloom; and the colour green, which helps bring peace and harmony in matters of the heart.

Chamomile
Chamomile is the most wonderfully soothing and calming of herbs and is therefore highly beneficial in the quest for restful sleep. Its value has

long been acclaimed, and there are records of its use going back to ancient times. It has the therapeutic ability to comfort the exhausted spirit, offering a gentle aromatic embrace at times of distress: a safe refuge. It opens up the ability to look at long-buried issues and bring a new understanding to them. This oil can bring about a renewed sense of order, by releasing built-up anger, tension, anxiety, and fear, which will help to bring about a state where rest and renewal can – at last – take place.

Embrace the soothing blue that chamomile brings to our energy field, as it helps us to voice our emotional needs and communicate our worries and fears, thus helping to bring about feelings of calm and gentle acceptance of life.

Frankincense

This relaxing oil is the protector of the spirit, reaching out into the realms of higher vibration and forming a protective field around us. It provides a sense of being elevated from the cares of our troubled mind – knowing that through contemplation and meditation, we can access higher aspects of ourselves to guide and support us through difficulties. It can bring about deeper breathing, a sense of being supported, and an ability to surrender, thus often releasing the stresses that cause sleeplessness.

The gentle violet colour released from frankincense oil is a true teacher of the spirit and penetrates our higher consciousness, prompting an awakening of our spiritual aspect.

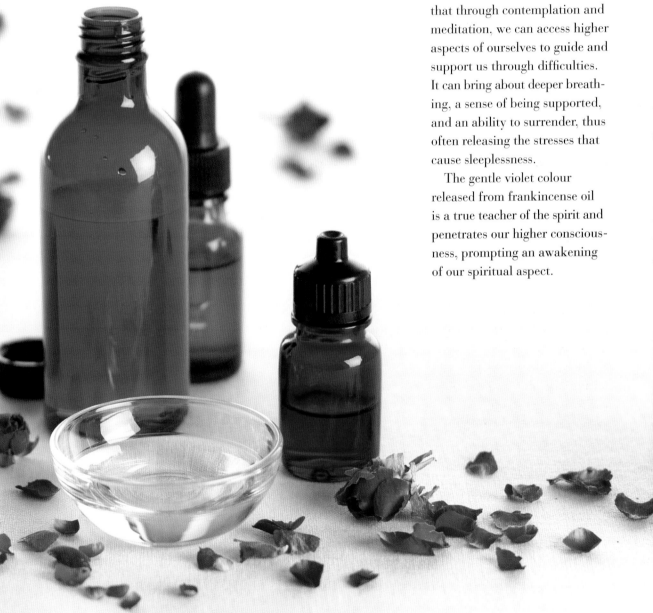

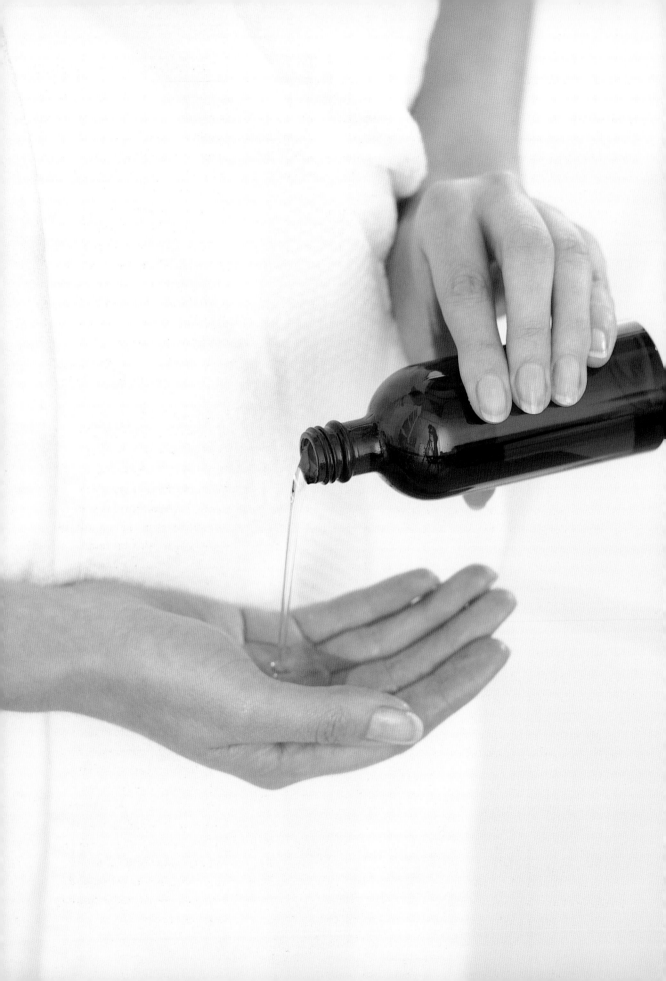

Jasmine

A highly prized, exotic, and beautifully perfumed oil, jasmine allows us to access both our masculine and our feminine qualities, bringing about a sense of reconciliation and balance. It releases us from the feeling of being "at war" with ourselves, which so often makes restful sleep impossible. We feel warmed by its wonderful fragrance and more able to look with honesty at the path we are treading, awakening self-confidence, the ability to make positive choices, and often improved quality of sleep.

Jasmine introduces the colours red and white to us, thus bringing a clearer understanding of our own actions and what motivates us. Red is the colour of life and white is the colour of the purity of the spirit. In order to live a life of harmony and balance, we are encouraged to welcome both in equal measure.

Marjoram

A deeply relaxing and fragrant herbal oil, marjoram is known for its soothing effects on muscular tension in the body, which can otherwise lead to wakefulness during the night. Marjoram also provides the warmth and comfort needed to heal and release feelings of grief or loss, bringing about a sense of deep peace and a connection through this peace to the whole of life. By encouraging the release of emotional obstructions, it also brings about a great renewal of creative energies – a sense of being able to flow through this wonderful life with ease.

The emotional qualities associated with marjoram are mirrored in its physical effects: it has the ability to stimulate blood flow by dilating the arteries and capillaries, thus producing feelings of warmth and stimulation.

We find the colours of blue and orange in the vibrational field of marjoram. Blue encourages us to look inwardly at our emotional needs, and orange finds a creative and joyful expression in these needs.

Rose

Rose oil encourages release of the most feminine aspects of ourselves – bringing us to a state of balance and peaceful sleep in the instances where this aspect has previously been either denied or put to one side. Its beautiful fragrance also allows

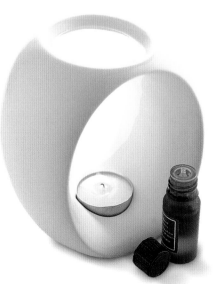

us, for a moment, to transcend earthly cares and rise to a more nourishing spiritual balance. Its beauty works on the heart, bringing the ability and worthiness to give, and receive, love unconditionally.

The colour vibration of rose oil is pink, which gently releases us into the higher consciousness of love for all. When we feel worthy of love ourselves, it is easy to share this powerful energy with others, bringing the gentleness and wonder of unity.

Sandalwood

When we feel that we have reached the end of our tether, bombarded by life's many demands, the rich and penetrating fragrance of this warm and rejuvenating oil can take us into a deeply relaxed state, enabling us to sleep soundly – after which we will feel more able to face life once more.

Sandalwood also releases the aggression within us and teaches that it is better to be united than divided, for we can all make use of each other's strengths and learn from each other's weaknesses. As well as helping us have compassion and understanding, sandalwood is deeply sedative and can induce drowsiness.

This oil introduces us to the colour violet, which helps to connect us to a higher wisdom, and the colour yellow, through which we can connect to, and develop a deeper understanding of, other people.

Aromatic massage

The gift of touch – and in particular massage – is of great benefit when you are feeling exhausted by many nights of disturbed sleep. And when combined with essential oils, it is a particularly effective way of easing you toward a restful night's sleep – at last.

Although there are a number of ways in which to use oils, massage is one of the most effective for insomnia or exhaustion, as the gentle care of a therapist or friend can be a really important form of both physical and emotional support. The massage on the following pages is very simple and is therefore something that anyone should feel confident enough to try on a friend. Having a third party who cares enough to want to help – along with the application of the therapeutic oils to the surface of the skin – is bound to have a positive effect. You could also – in theory – massage your own body, but there are areas of the back that would be hard to reach, making the process less rewarding. Allow about an hour to give, or receive, the massage suggested.

Setting the scene

The treatment room should be warm enough for the person receiving the massage to be comfortable, because the body loses heat quickly as it relaxes, and the use of oil on the skin can bring about even further heat loss. Plus, when at a low ebb, circulation tends to be sluggish, making the receiver particularly sensitive to the cold anyway.

Prepare the room, perhaps using scented candles and relaxing music. Essential oils need to be applied directly to the skin, so the person receiving the massage should remove all clothing. They should then lie comfortably on their front,

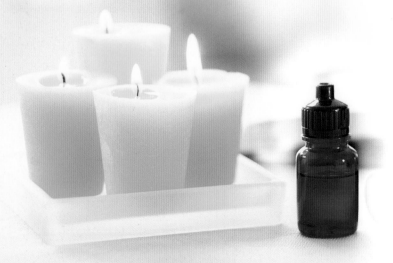

LIGHTS, CANDLES, ACTION
It is important that the person being massaged feels warm, comfortable, and completely at ease, so it may be worth lighting a few candles (beeswax are best) and putting on some gentle music before starting.

either on a mat on the floor or on a massage table. Next, cover the person with warm towels, which can be moved to the side as different areas of the body are worked on. You may even choose to place a hot water bottle at the receiver's feet. The person giving the massage should make sure that they can move freely and comfortably around the receiver, keeping the breathing as relaxed and even as possible.

Before applying any oils, give the entire back of the body (apart from the head) a stimulating rub. Start on the back, leaving the towels in place – and pay particular attention to the hands and feet in order to stimulate circulation. This is very relaxing and immediately removes any tension.

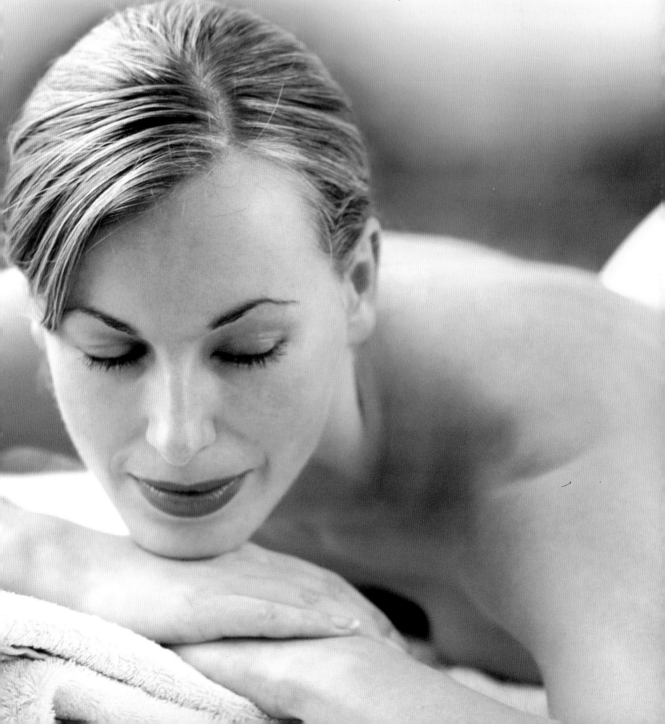

Getting down to business

Next, warm about one table-spoon of your "carrier oil" – the oil that is used to dilute the essential oils. Grapeseed oil or sweet almond oil work especially well for this purpose. Then add about five drops of your chosen essential oil to it (see pp. 104–107 for a choice). It is now time to introduce the oil to the skin.

The massage itself should be fairly gentle, yet firm enough to be effective. The movements should be smooth and circular. Concentrate on areas of muscle and soft tissue, and avoid working on bones, joints, and areas that are inflamed, tender, or bruised. Be led by your intuition and focus on the relaxing aspect of the massage more than technique: the healing properties of the oils will be more readily absorbed if the recipient is fully relaxed. Do, however, follow the guidelines on the following pages.

Giving a massage

An aromatic massage combines the nurturing power of touch with the healing power of scent. A weekly massage can help enormously in improving the condition of the muscles, releasing stresses and tensions before they become too deeply entrenched.

Start with the back

★ Start with large, firm circular movements on the back and shoulders. Be very gentle, however, around the neck.

★ Next, work some oil into the back of the arms, before covering the upper body with warm towels again. Use smaller movements when applying oils to these smaller parts of the body.

★ Then move down to the backs of the legs, feeling the body relax as the muscles relax. Use soft, sweeping movements on the calves, as these muscles can often be tense and sensitive.

★ Next, move on to the ankles and soles of the feet, before finishing the back of the body with a sweep up each leg, toward the heart.

...and now for the front

★ You can now ask your receiver to turn over onto their back if it is comfortable to do so. This time, you should work from the feet up to the head, so start by massaging oil into the feet and around the ankles.

★ Work up both legs, using stroking movements.

★ Next, work on each arm in turn. Hold the hand or wrist of the receiver with one hand, and use the free hand to apply the oil – working upward from the wrist. Then, work it into the hands and fingers.

★ Use small circular movements across the chest.

★ Use larger, circular movements on the stomach, working in a clockwise direction – up the right side; down the left – but avoiding too much pressure.

★ Then use small, gentle, circular movements around the face and jaw line. You can even sweep oil through the hair, working it firmly into the scalp. Hair is nourished and strengthened both by the stimulation of massage and by the oils themselves.

★ Return to the feet to finish the massage – holding them for a few moments, and breathing evenly. This is a wonderful way of ending the treatment.

Afterwards, it is important for both the giver and the receiver to drink lots of water and to rest. People often report having a good and restful night's sleep after a massage, especially if it takes place during the evening.

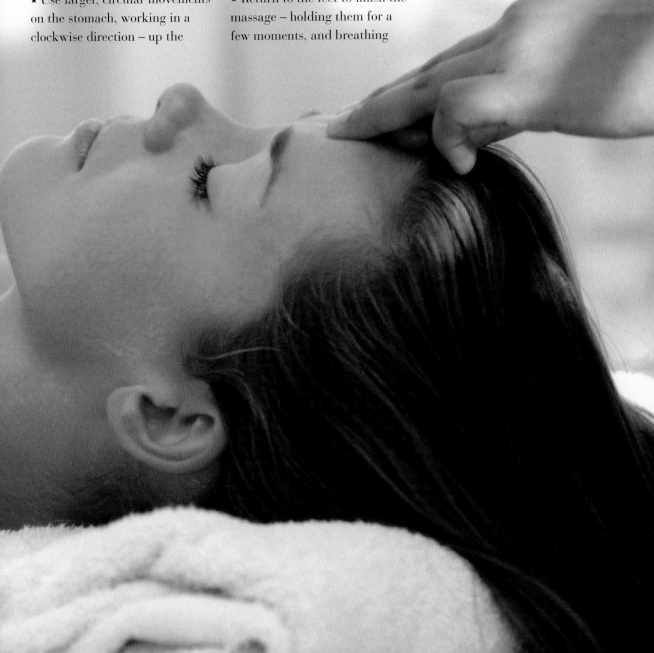

Massaging
the energy field

Massaging your energy field is a way of encouraging a healthy flow of energy around your body. When combined with relaxed and full breathing, it can realign your energy body with your physical body, creating a feeling of calm. It can be practised just before going to bed and also in the morning, if you are feeling sleepy or disorientated.

releasing of tensions. Be guided by your intuition, relaxing into the experience, to gain the maximum effects. But remember, you don't actually touch the body or the clothes; you should keep your hand 5–10cm (2–4in) above the surface.

Another method of introducing the healing qualities of aromatic oils is giving your aura, or energy field, a light massage. You can do this on yourself, remaining fully clothed if you wish, because you do not need contact with the skin – simply follow the guidelines on the following pages. It is a deeply relaxing exercise, which in addition to introducing the healing effects of essential oils, balances and redirects the energies of the body, giving rise to a clearing of the mind and a

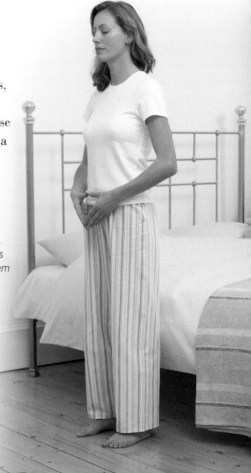

2 *Stand in a relaxed manner, slowing and deepening your breathing. Place the tip of your tongue lightly on the roof of your mouth, if it is comfortable to do so. Then touch the tips of your thumbs and fingers together, and allow them to rest in the area of the Tan Tien (lower abdomen; see p. 29).*

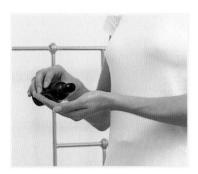

1 *Dilute two drops of your chosen oil in two drops of carrier oil, and rub over the palms of your hands.*

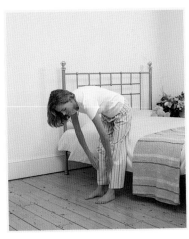

3 When your mind is quietly focused, start to bend forward, releasing your hands down your legs, 5–10cm (2–4in) from the surface of your body.

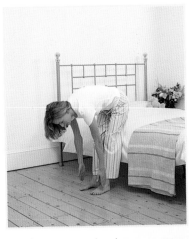

4 Now move your hands over your toes and round to your ankles, still avoiding contact with your body.

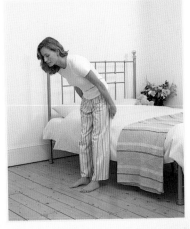

5 Then slowly move your hands up the back of your legs, over the buttocks...

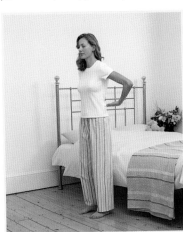

6 ...and as high up either side of your spine as you can without strain.

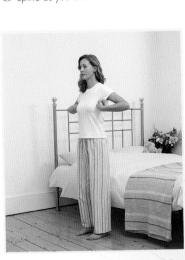

7 Now bring your hands forward to beneath the armpits (making loose fists).

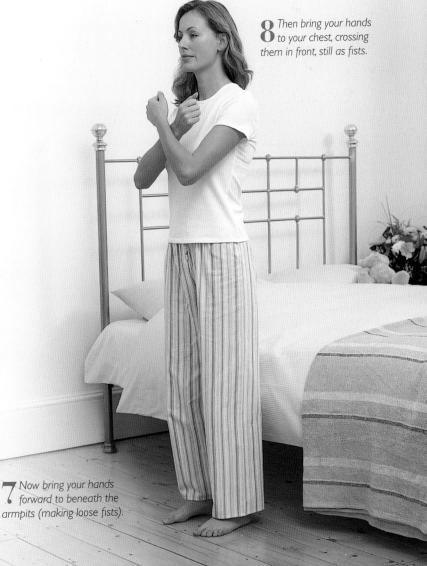

8 Then bring your hands to your chest, crossing them in front, still as fists.

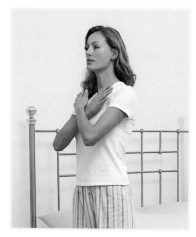

8 *Open your hands.*

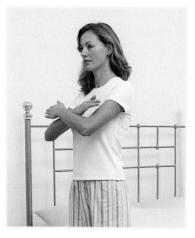

9 *Now draw your hands down the outsides of the opposite arms.*

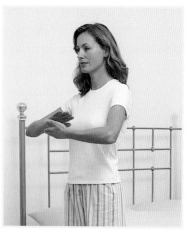

10 *Do this until the palms face one another at approximately chest-height.*

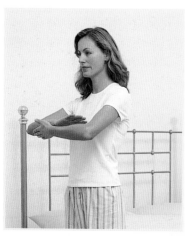

11 *Now push up the insides of your arms, until they cross over again.*

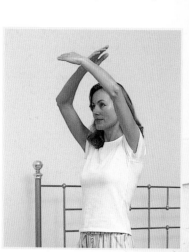

12 *Take your crossed hands over your head.*

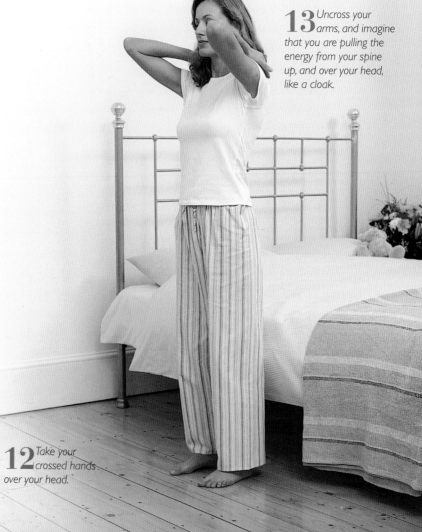

13 *Uncross your arms, and imagine that you are pulling the energy from your spine up, and over your head, like a cloak.*

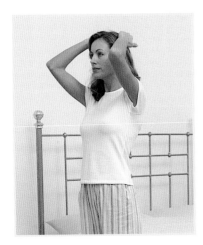

14 Continue pulling the energy up and over your head, now uncrossing your arms.

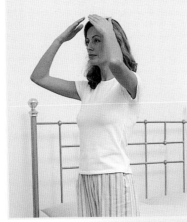

15 Gradually move your arms over the front of your head.

18 Return to the starting position of finger tips touching at the Tan Tien (lower abdomen) again, but this time with eyes closed.

Repeat this whole process three times, building up to nine times, and allowing the breath to flow freely throughout.

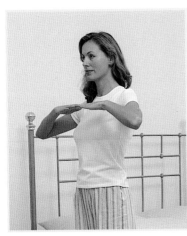

16 Start moving your hands down in front of your face

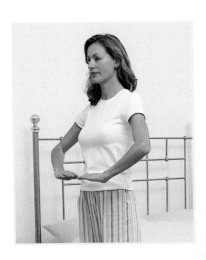

17 Continue moving your arms down the front of your body.

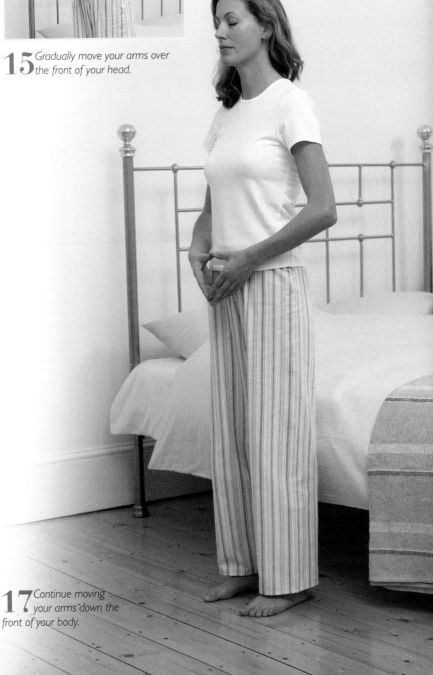

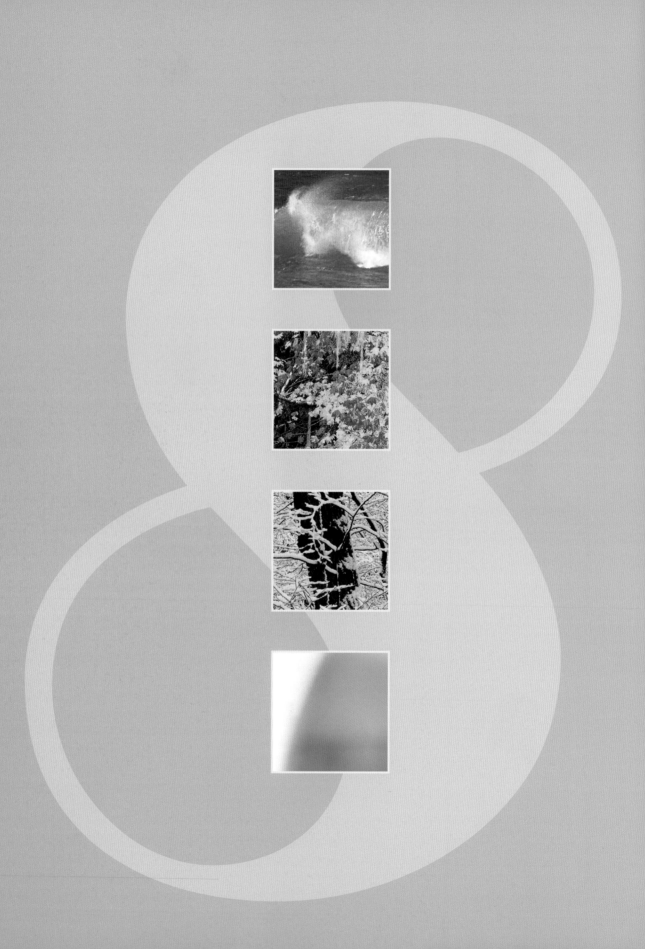

Chapter Eight

Healing with
COLOUR

Let the colours of the night

infuse your dreams — be rested

Colour therapy

Colour is an integral part of the world around us – appearing everywhere from the splendour of a sunset to brightly lit store windows. Whether we are aware of it or not, these colours have an influence over how we feel and have the power to uplift us and bring a smile to our faces. Colour therefore speaks to our senses and can have a therapeutic effect in our lives.

The energy that permeates our physical body and surrounds us has its own individual vibration, which resonates with the vibration of every colour or set of colours we come across. Someone in perfect health would have all the colours of the spectrum flowing throughout their aura in perfect balance. But, sadly, this is rarely seen, as the majority of us usually have some areas of life that need addressing.

The language of colour

By learning the language of colour, we can draw a little closer to understanding the workings of our own personal energy vibrations. Most of us have strong preferences for certain colours – often feeling an emotional response, for example, refusing to wear a certain colour or insisting that we paint the walls a particular shade. Often, we are attracted to a particular section of the spectrum – whether to the warm, earthy reds and oranges or to the balancing greens of nature.

Changing preferences

These preferences often change over time – an indication of changes taking place in our energy field. If we feel an aversion to a colour at a particular time, it can be an indication that this colour is "missing" or underdeveloped in our energetic make-up. As we progress into different states of awareness, we might well grow to like it in order to bring about increased balance.

Chakras

There are seven major energy centres, known as chakras, in our body (see right), and each of them vibrates at the same frequency as one of the rainbow colours – red, orange, yellow, green, blue, indigo, and violet. These chakras relate to particular areas of the body, and as they spin, they release colour into the aura. This is why the aura appears as fluctuating colours of light to people who are able to see it. However, certain conditions can cause them to be out of balance – underactive, overactive, distorted, or blocked and not functioning. Each of these is an indication that all is not well, and the use of colour as a gentle healing therapy is a way of bringing about a more even distribution of energy and thus more restful sleep for those who need it.

CROWN CHAKRA

Co-operation, service, self-confidence

THIRD EYE CHAKRA

Love, joy, deep awareness

THROAT CHAKRA

Intuition, truth, loyalty

HEART CHAKRA

Balance, trust

SOLAR PLEXUS CHAKRA

Intelligence, aspiration, courage

SACRAL CHAKRA

Sexuality, creativity, expression

BASE CHAKRA

Survival, action, drive, will

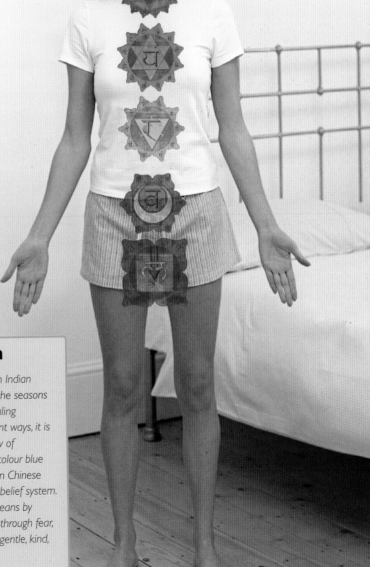

THE SEVEN CHAKRAS
This diagram shows the seven chakras of the body, each of which relates to a different colour vibration and encourages a different set of life qualities.

Varying colour symbolism

The seven colours relating to the chakras are based on Indian teachings, while the five relating to the elements and the seasons (see p. 45) are of Chinese origin. Although the two healing philosophies may initially seem to use colour in different ways, it is the symbolism that is important from the point of view of improving disturbed sleep patterns. For example, the colour blue signifies winter, the water element, fear and kindness in Chinese thinking, yet relates to the throat chakra in the Indian belief system. These are, however, related in that the throat is the means by which we give voice. If this is restricted or imbalanced through fear, the colour blue can soothe away the fears, leading to gentle, kind, and correct speech once again.

The 5colours

As already seen on page 45, Chinese health practitioners view the major organs of the body, the five elements, the five seasons of their calendar, and various emotional states in terms of five different colours. We can therefore make use of the vibrational aspect of colour in order to communicate with the energetic workings of the body and encourage sleep.

If we can bring about positive changes in the energetic imbalances through colour, then any imbalances in the body, leading to problems such as sleepless-ness, will gradually be corrected, too. Let us look at the colours in the Chinese healing model: the feelings that each promotes, and how each of them may be used

as a balancing vibration to prepare the body for quality sleep and recuperation.

Green

Visualize the colour green – the fresh green of change and new growth in springtime. This has a particular feeling of optimism, looking to the future with confidence and clarity.

It is the energy associated with the liver, and if this energy is in some way thwarted, it can lead to feelings of intense anger and frustration – the view that you are being left behind or left out of life. You may become irritable or defensive if this colour is out of balance, as your life is not progressing as you had hoped: your growth is being stunted, either by external circumstances or your inability to promote your own personal progress.

Consider, for a moment, how this relates to your own life and your own circumstances, and how the colour green, in this context, makes you feel. Think in particular about whether these feelings may be contrib-

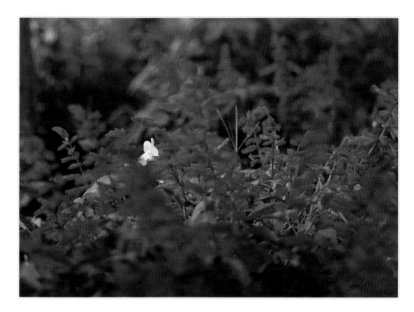

uting to feelings of stress or tension, which may be related to your inability to sleep.

Red

Bring to mind the colour red – an exciting vibrant red, pulsing with life and energy. It is the fire of the summer in all its glory and challenges you to awaken and be active in this life. It represents the blood of life, is the colour of the heart, and has the power to draw people together.

If this energy of the heart is not fully functioning and open, resentments and jealousies can easily arise, resulting in an attitude of meanness – a lack of desire to share with others, and feelings of loneliness or isolation. Love for self and for others is essential; out of these will arise a love for all of life. It is thought that imbalances in this energy – relating to fire – very commonly contribute to insomnia.

Consider the colour red in the context of your own life and outlooks, and examine how this colour makes you feel.

Yellow

We move on to the Chinese season of abundance – Indian summer (or harvest time) – and

the colour yellow. This is the colour of a gloriously warm and full sun, shining brightly upon everything. This is representative of the nurturing earth element. With this energy, we are able to gain nourishment from all experiences that come our way – digesting them and learning from them.

The vibrations of the colour yellow relate to the stomach, so a healthy balance brings a sense of happiness and belonging, which can help sleep to come more easily. If in any way inadequate, however, you will feel unable to "stomach" the situation in which you find yourself. It could be that this situation, far from nourishing you, is, in fact, draining your resources – physically, emotionally, or even financially. We have to learn to respect ourselves and our own needs before others will respect them.

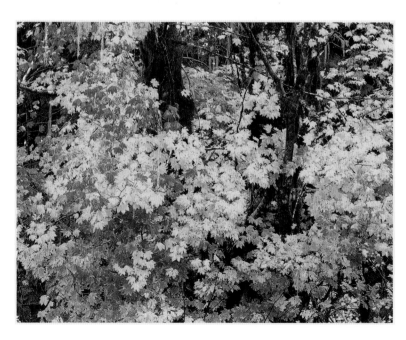

Consider how this relates to your own experiences, as you bring to mind the colour yellow.

White

Visualize the perfect white of freshly fallen snow. It provides a soft and gentle blanket – stilling noise and slowing down the hectic pace of daily activity. This is the colour of the metal element – strong and enduring. The vibration of white seeks to simplify and purify, illuminating the aspects of life that are truly essential. White signifies a time of peace, a time to re-evaluate and gather together vital resources. Through this, we can find qualities of great strength and courage – the courage not to grasp or hold on to what is not ours, and thus to release elements of our life that may be disturbing us emotionally at night-time.

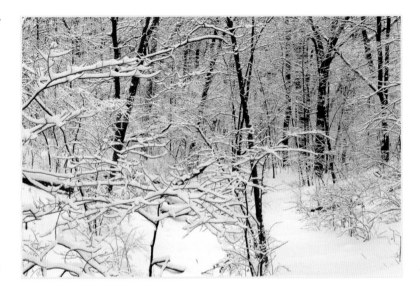

White is the colour associated with the lungs – the taking in and releasing of breath. When its energy is out of balance, we really feel the pains of life: we carry them with us, feeling sad, depressed, or betrayed, and we forget to lay down these burdens – holding on so tightly that we can barely breathe.

Consider the relevance of this energy to your own life, as you imagine yourself being bathed in pure white light.

Blue

Visualize yourself being transported up into a velvety blue night sky. Allow this colour to flood through you. Rich, deep blue to black is the colour of winter – symbolized by the water element. Consider, for a moment, the essential nature of water on this planet. Water is the basis for all of life. This colour's vibration teaches us the value of flowing with the waters of life, wherever they may take us, and accepting the changes to which this will inevitably lead, with grace and gentleness. Water seeks to show us our own reflection – often mirroring back to us those aspects of ourselves that we find difficult in other people. This gives us the chance to look deeply within and learn

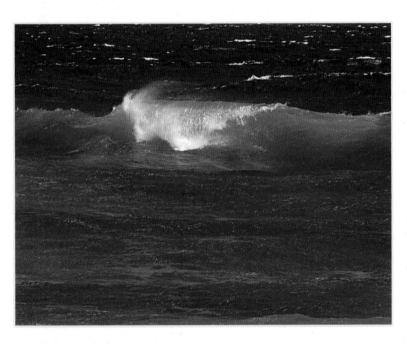

from what we see. Water can also be a strong force to be reckoned with, carrying us rapidly in its currents. A strong sense of the water element is an essential factor in helping us to drift off into sleep.

The water element is associated with the kidneys. When this aspect is out of balance, we can feel frightened by the forces of life. We may feel an undercurrent of anxiety as we go about our daily lives, leading to a feeling of complete exhaustion. We feel that life is fraught with danger and does not provide us with a place in which to rest. The kidney energy is viewed in Chinese medicine as the building ground for the other aspects: a good strong kidney energy will support you, while a depleted

one will leave you weak in your outlook toward life.

Imagine yourself immersed in a soothing blue. Feel the calm support it offers you, washing away complications and fear. Examine how this water energy relates to your life.

"Whooo" of blue

To further reinforce the healing energy that you wish to take to your kidneys, you may like to try an ancient Taoist healing contemplation. The healing sound for the kidneys is the sound "whooo" uttered gently, as if blowing a flame. Try the exercise that follows during times of sleeplessness. You can sit, stand, or lie down comfortably to do it. Close your eyes if it is easier for you:

★ Bring to mind the colour of a deep blue night sky – the healing colour for the kidney system. If you have difficulty in visualizing this colour, then simply intend it to be so and you will introduce the correct vibration.
★ Take your attention to the kidney area (in the lower back; see p. 65) and, in your mind's eye, flood it with your blue colour.
★ Take a deep breath, low down in the abdomen, and, as you exhale, breathe out with the sound "whoooo". Keep your attention on the kidneys and on the colour, and continue to breathe in this manner. You will probably feel the kidneys warming and strengthening.
• Repeat daily or simply when faced with a situation that provokes fear and anxiety.

The 5elements

The healing language of colour can be further explored by using an object of a certain colour (and element) to encourage its gentle vibrations to permeate your body. Contemplation is a powerful tool in itself, but when a coloured object from nature is incorporated, it becomes even more potent – helping your body, mind, and spirit to rebalance and realign.

Any severe or long-standing imbalance in the five elements – and therefore colours – can lead to insomnia. Thus each of the five elements has something to teach us about the personal challenges we need to face. We can use this understanding to bring about changes in our subtle bodies, through intro-ducing colour vibration.

Use your self-knowledge and intuition to decide which aspect – and therefore colour – needs to be worked with at any given time. It may be more than one, or your perception may even be that all the energies are somehow exhausted or depleted. If this is the case, then the colour blue, which represnts kidney

energy and the water element, is the one to concentrate on. If this is raised, then the others often follow suit. Alternatively, you could work through all the colours in turn. If you choose the latter option, it's best to use them in the following sequence: green, red, yellow, white, and blue. This will take you in the direction of growth and harmony, through the Chinese sequence of the "Five Elements", and will have a profoundly beneficial effect on your entire being.

The most difficult thing to do when trapped in the cycle of sleeplessness, exhaustion, and the need to keep fully function-ing, is, paradoxically, the thing that we most require – the

ability to relax. Relaxation is therefore a crucial aspect in the prevention and treatment of insomnia. The following exercise allows the mind and body to rest and relax by focusing on something harmonizing and positive.

Method

★ Choose something from nature that is the colour of the element you have chosen to work with. It could be a gemstone, a plant, or a flower. Make sure that you can sit, undisturbed, for a while.
★ Place your chosen item in front of you and study it.
★ Gaze into its depths, its textures, the way that the light catches it, its shape, its form. Breathe deeply and evenly as you continue to contemplate this item before you.
★ Without touching it, feel as though some part of you is reaching toward it and connecting with its essence. Enjoy this connection.
★ Now close your eyes and visualize your item – watch it in your mind's eye. Imagine it expanding until all you can

really see is its colour.

★ Continue breathing deeply and fully, and imagine that you are able to breathe this wonderful colour into your body. Feel the vibration of this colour as it fills your entire being.

★ Then feel that you are able to gently release this colour into the energy field throughout, and around, your body. Expand this gently until the whole of the room is full of this beautiful colour vibration. Relax into this sensation and enjoy the feelings of renewal that it brings. Rest in this energy.

★ When you feel ready to do so, imagine that you are able to gently draw this energy back toward your body. Continue to draw it back, focusing calmly on your abdominal region, as you gently breathe.

★ Imagine that you are able to inhale it into the Tan Tien – the seat of personal power in your lower abdomen (see p. 29). Relax, and focus your breathing on this centre.

★ When you are ready, have a gentle stretch, and give yourself a little time to come round. This time is just as important as the contemplation because it gives you the opportunity to assimilate the positive changes that you have introduced, making the exercise more effective and leaving you in a peaceful, rested state, ready to get a good night's sleep – at last.

5-ELEMENT CONTEMPLATION
Choose an object that evokes the element you want to work with.

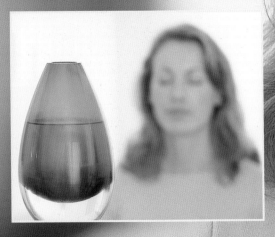

Index

Acknowledgements

A huge and heartfelt thanks to all the people who have had a hand in the writing and publishing of this book. The first thank you must go to my wonderful husband, Pete for his unswerving help and support, to my much-loved children – Henry, Emily and Lucy – and to my very special parents, all of whom have been a huge inspiration to me. Also to Steve and Jane who are so special and always seem to believe in me.

Thank you, too, to my enduring and inspired editor, Kelly, with whom I have shared many sleepless nights at the end of a computer. A big thank you to all my patient friends who have supported and encouraged me, albeit from afar, when I have been too busy to spend time with them. Thank you also goes out to Helen – a great and gifted healer – who, many years ago, told me that I was "worth something" and gave me the momentum I needed to turn my world around and follow my heart's desire. And finally, thank you to my many clients, who have all been teachers to me, as well as dear friends.

My hope is that everyone who reads this book will be able to proceed a little further along their path toward healing and awareness. We all have our own unique story to tell and our own journey to take, so enjoy your journey and the telling of your tale.